PRAISE FOR HOW TO BE HAPPY, HEALTH▪ ▪▪▪ WHOLE

"Meeting Victor five years ago was more than a blessing; it remains a treasure. This long overdue health masterpiece is not a run-of-the-mill book but a culmination of deep, thorough research: simple terms, easy read, and phenomenal results for anyone who values their health. Victor's integrity is what delayed this needed-to-be-written guide to a healthier life. He had to get it right and - wow - did he."

   - **Mark Januszewski,** Entrepreneur, Trainer and Best-Selling Author

"Wow! I went through Victor's book and was overall amazed! I didn't realize that things like junk food, caffeine, and sugar depleted magnesium! I'm adding magnesium to my regimen asap! Lately, I've slept more like 7-8 hours, and I have noticed that my appetite is more suppressed than when I was sleeping less. These couple of nuggets are amongst the midst of many, many more when it comes to our health! I'm now going to be using this book as a reference guide. Thanks, Victor! 'Health is wealth.'"

   - **Jermaine "Lead Monster" Steele**, Product Creation Coach and E-Commerce Specialist

"Victor's book is one of the most practical and easy-to-learn books on health and wellness. He lays it out in a very simple and powerful way - that keeps you reading. The usefulness of this book is incredible, and I look forward to using it as a go-to resource for health and nutrition. A brilliant piece of writing."

   - **Doctor Doug Firebaugh**, Coach, Speaker, Trainer, Entrepreneur, Author

"Wow, Victor explains what the number one master mineral is in this book and how we can avoid most health challenges by using it daily! "

   - **Jeff Altgilbers,** Entrepreneur, Coach and Mentor

"Imagine a world brimming with vibrant health, where knowledge empowers us to unlock our body's natural potential. That's the future Victor Dedaj's "How to Be Happy, Healthy and Whole" envisions, and it starts with a tiny but mighty mineral: magnesium!

Dedaj shines a light on magnesium deficiency as a hidden culprit behind many health struggles. But here's the exciting part: by understanding this essential mineral's role in our well-being, we can take charge! This book dives deep into how magnesium keeps our bodies functioning at their peak, from regulating muscles and nerves to supporting strong bones and a healthy heart. Dedaj equips you with the knowledge to boost your magnesium intake, exploring both dietary sources and strategic supplementation. Let's not be passive passengers on the road to health. Together, armed with this knowledge, we can become active participants in creating vibrant health for ourselves and those around us. Let's make optimal well-being the new standard, one magnesium-powered step at a time!"

- **Becca Dukes**, Director of Student Services and Trainer for the Institute of Wholistic Health, Certified Wholistic Health Coach, Functional Nutritional Consultant, Hostess of Daily with Doc and Becca

Contents

Foreword

In a world where health challenges are increasingly prevalent, the guidance of knowledgeable and compassionate individuals is more crucial than ever. This book, *How to Be Happy, Healthy and Whole*, authored by Victor Dedaj, stands as a beacon of wisdom and practical advice in the realms of health and nutrition.

Victor Dedaj is not just a Global Network Marketer in the health and nutrition sector; He is a Certified Holistic Health Coach with nearly two decades of dedication to this field. His journey began with a genuine concern for the well-being of his friends and family, sparked by articles highlighting the rampant health issues caused by poor dietary habits, over-medication, and nutrient deficiencies.

These insights fueled his passion for learning and sharing vital information on achieving better health. Victor's extensive experience and deep-seated commitment to helping others are evident throughout this book. He tackles the critical issues of our time—overconsumption of processed foods, inadequate intake of organic and nutritious foods, and the over-reliance on medications—providing readers with practical solutions to enhance their health. His approach is holistic, addressing not just the physical, but also the spiritual and mental well-being of individuals.

Having known Victor for many years, I have witnessed first hand his unwavering dedication to improving lives. His heart for helping others is not just professional but profoundly personal. He has touched many lives with his insights and support, guiding people towards healthier, more fulfilling lives. *How to Be Happy, Healthy and Whole* is more than a guide; it is a manifestation of Victor's mission to empower others with the knowledge and tools they need to thrive.

Whether you are at the beginning of your health journey or seeking to deepen your understanding, this book offers invaluable insights grounded in years of study and practical experience. I am confident that Victor's expertise and heartfelt commitment to holistic health will inspire and equip you to make meaningful changes in your life. May this book be your companion on the path to improved health and well-being.

With deep respect and gratitude,
Alan Newell,
20 year veteran, Christian Global Speaker and Trainer in the Direct
Sales, Affiliate Marketing Industry, Certified Holistic Health Coach
and Nutritionist

Introduction

Today, we are sicker than we have ever been. The truth is that the United States spends more on its healthcare system than any other country in the world, and the results have been horrible. One of the problems is that very little is spent on preventative health, and the majority is spent on treating sickness. Remember, an ounce of prevention is worth a pound of cure. They say the best way to treat cancer is to prevent it from happening in the first place. We spend 97.5% of our healthcare budget on individual treatment, while we only spend 2.5% on prevention. It is much better not to get cancer or heart disease than to try to treat those diseases when you get them. Speaking of cancer, only 33 percent of people living with cancer are said to be "cured" (that is, they have a five-year event-free survival), while only 7 percent avoid developing another cancer during the next 20 years.

Fewer people today are dying from heart attacks (mostly due to prompt treatments in emergency rooms and hospitals), but more people have suffered at least one heart attack than in the past.

One out of every five deaths is attributed to poor diet. Most of the top ten causes of death (e.g., heart disease, cancer, diabetes, Alzheimer's disease) are also linked to the downstream effects of having a bad and poor diet. So, eating a bad and poor diet is making many people very sick.

We are told not to smoke (which is a good thing). However, we are not told that we are severely deficient in nutrients, which is causing all kinds of health issues. When we get sick, we expect to get a magic pill from our doctor, hoping it will magically solve our problems. It doesn't happen. The medicines we are given usually only treat the symptoms but rarely treat the underlying cause. That is why people have been on medications for decades. The underlying condition is not addressed, and other health issues arise. Then, more meds are given, and people often wind up taking five to ten medications, all of which have various side effects. You will never meet someone who says, "I am on ten medications a day, and I feel great!"

When you take your dog to the vet and there is a problem with the dog, one of the first questions the veterinarian will ask is, "What are you feeding this dog?" Contrast that to when you go see your doctor when you are sick. How often does the doctor ask, "What are you feeding your kid?" or "What are you feeding yourself?" You are more likely to be asked, "What kind of meds are you taking?" "The first step is to give up the illusion that the primary purpose of modern medical research is to improve Americans' health most effectively and efficiently. In our opinion, the primary purpose of commercially funded clinical research is to maximize financial return on investment, not health." - John Abramson, M.D., Harvard Medical school

The human species is the only species with "experts." We are also the only species with a chronic disease epidemic.

We are eating processed foods, ultra-processed foods, and genetically modified foods that are usually devoid of nutrients and fiber and loaded with junk. Your body is crying for nutrients, and most of the foods you are eating are not providing the nutrients your body wants. The S.A.D. (Standard American Diet) is nowadays mostly C.R.A.P. (Completely Refined and Processed) diet.

Did you know that kids who eat lots of processed food don't do as well in school as kids who eat far less processed foods?

Unfortunately, most people do not get proper information about the importance of nutrition and why they need more nutrients in their diets.

The vast majority of schoolchildren are not taught or exposed to nutritional education while they are in school.

Doctors spend little time in medical school learning about nutrition or nutritional supplementation. Their focus in medical school is on studying diseases, not wellness.

Most doctors don't understand the power of food and the power of nutrition and supplements.

Only twenty-eight percent of medical schools have a formal nutritional curriculum. Eighty percent of the medical curriculum is underwritten by Big Pharma.

Medical students, on average, receive about twenty contact hours of instruction in nutrition during four years of medical school, which is about 0.25% of the time spent in class. This is why you usually don't get good nutritional advice from your doctor. He probably did not learn it in medical school. Think about it this way: if you spent all those years in medical school and spent so little time teaching nutrition, you would probably think nutrition is not that important. By the way, I am not telling you to stop going to see your doctor. I d recommend that you don't give your doctor all the power over you

4

and don't treat him like a god, which is what a lot of people do. Doctors do make mistakes sometimes. And it is fine to get a second opinion if your doctor urges you to get an operation and you are not sure if you should do it. I recommend trying to find one who has knowledge of nutrition and whose first response is not to prescribe drugs for you automatically.

Remember, many doctors used to say that cigarettes were healthy and fine to use. There used to be ads showing doctors smoking. Dentists used to study nutrition in dentistry until 1947, and then dental schools stopped the nutrition classes.

Since 2000, we have eaten less in the U.S. and exercised more, yet we have become more obese.

The US ranks 47th in the world in life expectancy. We have five percent of the world's population and spend about fifty percent of the world's medical care spending. We have the most expensive medical system in the world, but we don't have the best medical system in the world. The United States ranks 69th in world health. Men lie, and women lie, but numbers don't lie. If we were doing well and we were getting a really good bang for the buck for all that we spend on medical care, then the US would not rank 47th in life expectancy.

Many diseases that barely existed a hundred years ago, such as diabetes, cancer, heart disease, and Alzheimer's, have exploded in the last sixty years.

President Richard Nixon declared the "War on Cancer" in 1971. We were promised by the medical establishment a cure for cancer by 1976. However, cancer rates continue to increase in our society nearly five decades later.

We need to ask why this is happening. Why are things not getting better but worse regarding our health? People are getting cancer in their twenties, which was almost nonexistent fifty years ago. Not only has there been a spike in obesity and diabetes among adults, but it has also spiked among teenagers and children as well. Fatty liver disease used to only happen to alcoholics. Now, it has become rampant among people who aren't alcoholics and has been given the name nonalcoholic fatty liver disease.

Dr. Mark Hyman writes in his book Food Fix, "Our diet is the number one cause of death, disability, and suffering in the world. Our food has dramatically transformed over the last hundred years, and even more radically over the last forty years, as we have eaten a diet of increasingly ultraprocessed foods made from a handful of crops (wheat, corn, soy)." Dr. Hyman continues, "Chronic disease is now the biggest single threat to global economic development. Lifestyle-caused diseases such as heart disease, diabetes, and cancer now kill nearly fifty million people a year, more than twice as many as die from infectious diseases. Two billion people go to bed overweight and eight hundred million go to bed hungry in the world today. One in two Americans and one in four teenagers have pre-diabetes or type 2 diabetes."

They say that insanity is doing the same thing repeatedly and expecting different results. Things will be bad if you keep doing the same things that have led to this health debacle. Some things need to change.

Despite all the bad news, there is hope and light at the end of the tunnel. Once you start taking care of your body and giving it the things it needs to function well, it can start recovering and work well.

More doctors have learned the importance of nutrition for health and are getting the word out through books and videos on YouTube and other channels. They all admit that they learned little about nutrition in medical school and later learned just how important nutrition was. I have quoted a number of doctors in this book.

The truth is most people don't know what to do. I see many people around me suffering health wise, and I know they can be doing better. My desire is to see you, your family, and your friends live a better, happier, and healthier life. It is definitely possible!

We will go over the things that have wrecked and destroyed our health over the past seventy years, and we will also go over what we can do to have good health and a great lifestyle.

Chapter 1
American/Western Diet

Hippocrates said, "Let food be thy medicine and medicine be thy food."

There are over six-hundred different poor health conditions linked to nutritional deficiencies. The Standard American Diet is also known as S.A.D., and it is really sad.

Over the last sixty years, the American diet has drastically changed. People were encouraged to change their diet to become low-fat and high-carb. All fats, such as butter and cheese, were demonized. The thinking was that if it has fat, it must make you fat and more susceptible to heart attacks.

What has resulted from this switch to a high-carb, low-fat diet? A huge increase in cardiovascular diseases and heart attacks, as well as an increase in obesity and diabetes. These diseases were rare in 1900. In 1900, Americans consumed far less sugar. They also consumed very little vegetable/seed oils back then. What we eat today goes against what we ate for most of human history, and we are paying the price for it.

Dr. David Perlmutter writes in his book *Drop Acid*, "It makes sense that our DNA works best with an ancient diet. For more than 99 percent of the time we have existed on this planet, we have eaten a diet much lower in refined carbohydrates, higher in healthful fat and fiber, and much more nutrient-dense in general than the diets we eat today. And we didn't eat processed or fast foods then, either: we ate what we could find in nature. In fact, our modern-day Western diet works against our DNA's ability to protect health and longevity. And we experience the consequences of this mismatch every day."

Many people don't understand the power of the Compound Effect, which can work for you or against you. Small, little changes over time can lead to big, dramatic results. A penny doubled over a few days becomes $0.02, $0.04, $0.08, and $0.16, and it seems like very little happens in the beginning. However, after thirty-one days, that penny doubled to $10,737,418.24.

You can have two men who have similar weight and a similar build. One person starts eating lots of terrible, unhealthy junk food and doesn't exercise at all. The second person begins eating healthy food and a healthy diet and exercises regularly and lifts weights. After a week, the two men look pretty much the same, and nothing seems to have changed. Three years later, the first guy has put on a lot of weight, has less energy, and is starting to develop some health issues. The second guy lost some weight, has more energy, has developed some muscles, and is overall healthy. The compound effect negatively affected the first man and positively affected the second man.

If you had a heart attack after eating a McDonald's Big Mac, you would probably never eat a Big Mac. However, when you eat your first Big Mac, nothing bad happens to you, so you think it's ok and enjoy the taste of the Big Mac. If you consistently eat Big Macs for years, your body will start to feel the detrimental health effects of eating all those Big Macs.

SNAP (Supplemental Nutrition Assistance Program) households spend about ten percent of their dollars on soda and sugary drinks. That is about three times as much as they spend on milk.

Believe it or not, the USDA guidelines state that for two-year-olds, up to 10% of their diet can be added sugar. That is a recipe for diabetes later on in life.

There are many civilizations where people have lived very healthy lives. Once they are exposed to the Western Diet and try the same foods we eat here in the United States, they start getting sicker and getting diseases that did not exist in their civilization before.

Sixty percent of Americans have at least one or more chronic illnesses, and forty percent have two or more chronic illnesses. Clearly, the medical system is not working.

Many companies will put harmful ingredients in their products in the United States, and they don't put the same product in other countries because those countries don't allow those ingredients. For example, Kellogg's Froot Loops have some harmful color additives like Red 40, Yellow 5, Yellow 6, and Blue 1, which Froot Loops do not have in Canada. Why doesn't Kellogg's also take those products out of Froot Loops in the United States? This goes on with a lot of products. The US version of many foods will have more ingredients than the European version because European countries don't allow certain compounds and ingredients because of health concerns.

The following chemicals and substances are found in many foods in the United States that you won't find in Europe because of health concerns: potassium bromate, titanium dioxide, brominated vegetable oil, propylparaben, and azodicarbonamide. People in Europe live longer than people in the United States, and the rates of chronic disease are also lower there. Could these chemicals and substances that are banned in Europe be one of the reasons Europeans live longer than Americans?

The United States is 4% of the world's population, yet we were 16% of the deaths from COVID. One of the reasons that happened is because of our compromised health, which is worse than in much of the rest of the world, which made us more susceptible to COVID. For many decades, we have been told that we need to lower our salt intake because it can lead to high blood pressure, heart disease, stroke, and other health issues. There is no scientific data behind these recommendations. In fact, a low salt diet can lead to a whole bunch of issues, such as increased heart rate. The countries of France, Japan, and South Korea all have low rates of high blood pressure, coronary heart disease, and death as a result of cardiovascular disease. These three countries also eat a high-salt diet. Canada and Switzerland have low rates of death due to stroke even though they eat a high salt-diet. Many countries that eat the most salt also have long life expectancies. Japan has the highest life expectancy in the world. Latvia has about half the salt intake of Japan (7 grams versus 13 grams), and Latvia has a death rate that is ten times greater than Japan. Salt is not the problem. Look at stuff such as sugar and seed oils instead.

You also need salt to make stomach acid, which is essential as stomach acid is required to digest nutrients. People have been told for decades to eat more grains because they are healthy. Grains cause inflammation, which can lead to S.I.B.O. (Small Intestinal Bacterial Overgrowth), obesity, hormonal imbalances, type-2 diabetes, and many other illnesses.

Chapter 2
Vitamin and Mineral Deficiencies

The truth is that most diseases are caused by vitamin and mineral deficiencies. Most people are severely deficient in various vitamins and minerals, and those deficiencies lead to various illnesses and diseases.

Two-time Nobel Prize winner Dr. Linus Pauling said that you could trace every sickness and disease to a nutritional deficiency. Colloidal minerals are the best because they are over 95% absorbable by the body. This is why it's a good idea to eat plants, as we can get colloidal minerals from them.

Unfortunately, many doctors and many other people tell the public that they can get all the vitamins and minerals from their diet. That is absolutely false. The government has known since 1936 that we can't get all the nutrients we need from our diet and that our soil is deficient in nutrients. US Senate Document #264, written in 1936, states, "The soil is so nutritionally deficient of minerals that it will NOT supply the necessary nutrition for good health." That was almost 90 years ago, in 1936. The soils have gotten worse and more nutritionally deficient since then.

No matter how healthy your diet is, even if it is all organic and has no processed foods, it won't give you all the nutrients you need. Many people who are misled into believing this are paying the price by getting sick and dying early as a result of this. If these people had supplemented to make up for their deficient nutrients, they would be healthier and live longer. Being deficient in the mineral calcium alone can lead to about 150 different diseases. Altogether, nutritional deficiencies can lead to about 900 different diseases. Broccoli has 85% fewer nutrients than it did 80 years ago. Many other fruits and vegetables have 40 to 90 percent fewer nutrients than they did 70 to 80 years ago. There is no way you can eat all the fruits and vegetables necessary for your optimal health because of the scarcity of nutrients these days, and you are not going to find too many people who are going to eat 50 to 60 pieces of fruits and vegetables a day to do it.

So what can you do instead of eating 50 servings of fruits and vegetables? You need to supplement. Make sure to get good quality supplements. Don't buy store brands like the national pharmacy chains, as those tend to have very little absorption. Basically, you are throwing your money away. It's not what you consume that matters; it's what you absorb. Make sure you get supplements that are absorbable. Don't be penny-wise and pound-foolish. Also, make sure you are eating really good and less of the cheaper processed food. Try to eat more organic food if possible. If you worry that it will cost more, there is a saying that you should pay the farmer now or the doctor later. The choice is yours.

One thing to keep in mind about supplements: although I stress supplementing is very important, that does not give you license to keep a very unhealthy diet. You can't out-supplement a bad diet. If you supplement but eat lots of processed and junk food, you will eventually have health issues. You need to both supplement and eat healthy food.

Your body needs 60 minerals, 16 vitamins, 12 amino acids, and 2-3 essential fatty acids. Altogether, that is 90 nutrients. Look at the foods and the nutritional information you get from them. Once you look at the nutritional information, you will see that you are not getting all the nutrients you need, which is why you will need to supplement.

Minerals are about ⅔ of your body's nutritional needs. Plants and animals can't make minerals. It must be in the soil. Sometimes, pesticides and herbicides prevent minerals from going to the plant. Minerals are also crucial because vitamins can't work without them. That is another reason to ensure your body gets all the necessary minerals.

Plants can sometimes make vitamins. While it is growing, the plant receives nutrients from the soil and energy from the sunlight. The plant will use the energy to convert its nutrients. This will cause the plant to grow and produce more enzymes, phytonutrients, and compounds. Vitamins will naturally occur as a consequence of this action.

Farmers understand vitamin and mineral deficiency because they can't insure their animals. There is no Blue Cross and Blue Shield or United Healthcare insurance for cows, pigs, chickens, or horses. Farmers have to make sure that their animals don't get sick, so they give them enough vitamins and minerals each day to make sure they don't get sick. The farmer does not want to spend $50,000 for an operation for his animal, so he ensures the animals get all the vitamins and minerals they need.

The question is, "Why don't we do the same things with humans?" There is no focus on making sure humans get all the vitamins and minerals they need each day to keep them healthy like they do with animals. It makes you wonder why.

Chapter 3
The Pharmaceuticals (Big Pharma)

One huge culprit in terms of people being sick is Big Pharma. What many people don't realize is that Big Pharma does not want people to be healthy. They only make money when people are sick. As long as you are healthy, they make no money. All the Big Pharma companies admit they are in business to make a profit. That is all they care about. The more sick people there are, the more money they make.

We do not have a health care system. We have a sick care system—the ones who profit from this are Big Pharma, Big Agriculture, and Big Food.

In the 2020 DGAC (Dietary Guidelines Advisory Committee), 95% of the committee members had at least one tie with a pharmaceutical or food company. Half of the committee members had 30 such ties. The companies with the most frequent and durable connections to the committee included Kraft, Kellogg, Abbott, General Mills, Dannon and Mead Johnson.

It turns out that 9 of the 20 experts (45%) on the 2025 Dietary Guidelines Advisory Committee were found to have had conflicts of interest in the pharmaceutical, weight loss, food, or beverage industries during the last five years.

Big Pharma contributes nearly ⅔ of the FDA's budget, so you can bet the government agency often goes easy on them. Every single pharmaceutical company spends more on marketing than on research and development.

Meds don't cure diseases but only treat the symptoms. Twenty percent of people in the US over the age of 65 take at least five different medications. Taking more than five pills a day is associated with an increased risk of mortality.

The FDA (Food and Drug Administration) should be called the Federal Drug Administration. Only about 7% of the FDA's budget deals with food, and about 93% deals with drugs. The FDA commissioners usually wind up going to work for the pharmaceuticals once they leave the FDA.

Almost 50% of the FDA's budget comes from user fees paid by pharmaceuticals to get their drugs or medical devices approved. And 75% of the agency's drug division is funded by the pharmaceutical industry from those fees.

Pharmaceutical and health product companies spent over $372 million to lobby Congress and federal agencies in 2022. The $372 million outspent all other industries and made up over half of the lobbying efforts in the health sector.

Big Pharma and Big Food work together. Big Pharma owns some of the Big Food companies.

Corporate Dietetic Organizations get 90 percent of their funding from Big Food, so they constantly exonerate processed foods and sugars.

Pharmaceuticals spend tons of money on advertising.

Pharmaceutical companies like Novo Nordisk also give lots of money to civil rights groups and obesity lobby organizations. These groups claim the donations do not influence them. Can we really believe that? What happens is that these groups influence their members to take the meds made by these pharmaceutical companies.

Fifty percent of news funding is paid by pharmaceutical companies. That is why you rarely see anything negative on the news about pharmaceuticals or pharmaceutical drugs. It is also why you rarely hear anything good said about vitamins and minerals on the news. You will see tons of commercials about pharmaceutical drugs, but rarely commercials talking about how great healthy vitamins and minerals are.

A study done by researchers at Pennsylvania State University found that from 2013 to 2022, 826,313 of more than 1.4 million eligible doctors received more than 85 million payments from American pharmaceutical drug makers and device manufacturers. That is about 57 percent of the doctors and the total payments to them added up to about $12.1 billion. Some of the money went to consulting and non-consulting fees such as speaking fees. These doctors were also given travel and lodging, entertainment, education, food and beverages, charitable donations and grants, and honoraria. This can lead to a conflict of interest with the types of medications doctors prescribe to patients, as well as a loss of trust in the independence of the medical profession.

The biggest payments went to orthopedic surgeons, psychiatrists, neurologists, and cardiologists.

Orthopedic surgeons received $1.36 billion, while psychiatrists and neurologists received $1.32 billion. Cardiologists received $1.29 billion.

The United States is not the only country where this happened. In Australia, pharmaceutical companies paid about AU$ 21.7 million from 2019 to 2022 to over 6,500 doctors to promote their products and services.

The American Diabetes Association, the American Heart Association, and the American Cancer Society make millions and millions of dollars each year from the diseases their association covers. They have no incentive to have cures for these diseases as they make so much money off of it. If the diseases are cured, then they won't make money. That is why they recommend you take pharmaceutical drugs, often from their sponsors. If you look at the web site for the American Diabetes Association for corporates sponsors, you will see companies like Pfizer, Merck, and Novo Nordisk (among others) that make pharmaceutical drugs.

Six in ten adults in the US have a chronic disease. Four in ten adults have two or more chronic diseases.

Not only do drugs have all kinds of side effects, but they also drain us of nutrients, which help make us sicker.

There is a place in medicine for drugs. If I need to be operated on and they need to open me up during the surgery, I want an anesthetic to knock me out during surgery. I don't want to be awake while they are cutting me up.

There have been a good number of drugs that have helped a lot of people. I am not denying that.

The problem is that doctors are taught in medical school to treat almost all cases with drugs. Very little attention is paid to nutrition in medical schools. Doctors may get a three-hour course or something on nutrition and very little else. That is why many doctors have little understanding of nutrition and how important vitamins and minerals are for health.

Big Pharma understands that there is no money in vitamins, which is why they often sponsor bogus studies showing that vitamins don't help or are even dangerous. One thing that is done sometimes in these studies is that they test the synthetic form of the vitamins, which is very different from taking the natural form of the vitamin. I would recommend staying away from the synthetic form of vitamins. You often don't get the benefits you would from the natural form of the vitamin.

Big Pharma knows that a patient cured is a patient lost. It makes money when people get sick.

What some people don't understand is that drugs don't cure anything. They never have, and they never will. What drugs do is that they mask the symptoms, but the underlying symptoms remain.

Another big problem with taking drugs is that they often have nasty side effects. Sometimes you have to take another drug to offset the fact that you are allergic to the drug you are taking.

Vitamins and minerals don't have the side effects drugs do.

Dr. Robert Lustig, in his book *Metabolical*, writes, "Despite the billions of dollars poured into pharmaceutical research, no drug can fix any of these eight pathologies because drugs are not nutrients. Only real food works. In fact, Big Pharma is adept at covering up this subterfuge by advertising directly to the consumer, pretending the symptoms are the disease. They're not." He also says, "Physical activity is a useful adjunct, but you can't outrun a bad diet."

The third leading cause of death in the United States is prescription drugs and medical errors. This is criminal, yet the government does nothing to punish the companies that make these drugs that are killing people. Why are doctors being trained in medical school to prescribe drugs that often have harmful side effects and wind up killing people?

I don't blame the doctors. Most doctors go into medicine because they want to make a difference in people's lives and help people. I have many friends who are doctors and I know they really care about their patients.

A lot of people don't know that the liver, which cleanses your body of toxins, sees medical drugs as poisons and works to get rid of them. That is why when you are prescribed a drug, you are prescribed high doses so that the liver can't get rid of all of it. It's really messed up that the medical community prescribes drugs that are considered poisons by our bodies.

One hopeful note is that more doctors seem to be aware of naturopathic ways of healing people. Rest assured, they are not learning this in medical school, but they learned it elsewhere. A good number of them write books and put out videos focusing on diet and nutrition instead of drugs to help people become healthy.

It is funny they refer to healing people in natural ways without drugs as "Alternative Medicine," even though this was the way medicine was practiced for thousands of years. The real "Alternative Medicine" is the allopathic way doctors are taught in med school, where they treat the condition by giving meds that cover the symptoms. Also, they focus on one part of the body. On the other hand, Wholistic practitioners focus on the whole person as they know that everything is interrelated in the body.

Almost all cancer doctors will recommend chemotherapy for people who have cancer. What is the problem with chemotherapy? First of all, it is made from mustard gas, the deadly weapon used in World War II. Chemotherapy not only kills the cancer cells, it kills the good cells as well, and the person's immune system is destroyed. When your immune system is destroyed, you are susceptible to just about everything. Chemotherapy will also destroy your nutrients, which will hurt your immune system.

Another problem is that the underlying reason for the cancer is not taken care of in chemotherapy. Chemotherapy sometimes leads to cancers in other parts of the body. Say you eat a very nutrient-deficient diet and don't supplement your diet. That may be one cause of cancer. If you don't change that, you will likely get sick again and may get cancer again in the future. It is one reason cancer is often recurring in many people.

One of the reasons Big Pharma hates vitamins and minerals is that there is no money in them.

Can you believe that the FDA states that vitamins and minerals can't cure disease and that only drugs can cure disease? That is totally ridiculous. Drugs only mask symptoms. They don't cure. This is why you will never see vitamin and mineral supplements state that they cure any disease. They will state that it may support liver health or blood sugar support, for example.

Often, drug companies become aware of really terrible side effects of the drugs they bring to the market, and they hide it from the public.

Merck, in November 2007, announced that it would pay $4.85 billion to end thousands of lawsuits that were filed against the painkiller Vioxx that was used to treat arthritis. At the time, it was believed to be the largest drug settlement. And, of course, they paid without admitting guilt or fault. Vioxx was pulled off the market in 2004.

According to an article published in the Journal of American Medicine (JAMA) in 2008, Merck was aware of the dangers of Vioxx but withheld the information from federal officials and played down the number of deaths associated with the drug. Merck was also aware that people who were at risk for Alzheimer's disease in

17

two clinical trials for Vioxx had a death rate three times that of the participants who took the placebo.

FDA Senior Investigator Dr. David Graham said that before Vioxx was removed from the market in 2004, it may have hurt hundreds of thousands of patients and killed about a third of them.

A study was published in May 2006 by McGill University Health Center that appeared in the Canadian Medical Association Journal, almost two years after Merck voluntarily withdrew Vioxx from the market. The findings showed that 25% of the patients who had heart attacks while taking Vioxx suffered them within two weeks of taking the drug.

A study that was published in the Lancet suggested that Vioxx could have been responsible for between 88,000 and 140,000 additional cases of serious coronary heart disease in the United States.

In May 2024, Pfizer quietly agreed to settle 10,000 cancer lawsuits that accused Pfizer of hiding cancer risks brought about by their anti-heartburn medication Zantac.

In the 19th century and the early part of the 20th century, the medical marketplace was much different than it is today. You had naturopaths, homeopaths, osteopaths, chiropractors, allopaths (MDs), and herbalists all competing for patients as well as territory and recognition.

The Flexner Report changed medicine here in the United States in the early part of the 20th century. Flexner did a five-year study of medical schools on their use of drugs and brought the report to Carnegie. Carnegie and Rockefeller then funded the medical schools to prescribe drugs. The Rockefellers and Carnegies pretended to be concerned with public safety and set a standard of educational competence for all medical schools. What they really wanted to do was dominate the medical marketplace and get rid of the competition (Homeopaths, Herbalists, Chiropractors, Acupuncturists, Osteopaths, and Naturopaths). Many of the homeopathic and chiropractic schools closed down.

Thirty percent of the medical schools and hospitals at the beginning of the 20th century were Homeopathic ones. By 1920, eight years after the Flexner report came out, all of the Homeopathic Hospitals and Schools were closed.

While working for the Yerkes Primate Research Center in Atlanta, Dr. Joel Wallach discovered that Cystic Fibrosis was not just a human disease. Animals could get it, too, and he showed that a

Rhesus Monkey could get cystic fibrosis (CF). If the pregnant mother was deficient in the mineral selenium, then her babies would be born with cystic fibrosis. To thank him for these groundbreaking and amazing findings, Dr. Wallach was let go from his job. Why was that? First, he showed that Cystic Fibrosis was not genetic, which the entire medical world believed. He also showed that the treatment was simply supplementing with the mineral selenium, and there is no money to be made with selenium preventing cystic fibrosis.

In 1987, in Wilkes vs. the AMA (American Medical Association), the AMA was found guilty by Judge Susan Getzendanner of an illegal conspiracy against the chiropractic profession and of orchestrating a campaign of slander and mudslinging of negative PR as well antitrust behavior over many years against the Chiropractic profession. The decision said that the largest physicians' group in the nation led a boycott of physicians "to contain and eliminate the chiropractic profession." The Court awarded $25 million to the Chiropractic Association as compensation.

Pharmaceutical drugs are big money. Statin drugs had a market size of $15 billion in 2023. The pharmaceuticals are raking in big money.

There is very little research done on vitamins, minerals, or herbs. Anyone could make it if a mineral was shown to cure lung cancer. You could not put a patent on it like you could do with a pharmaceutical drug. There is no incentive to research vitamins and minerals because you can't make money off them if you discover they can help treat and cure diseases.

The incidence of disease has skyrocketed since the pharmaceutical and allopathic doctors took over medicine.

The advances in medicines have not been in cures for heart disease, cancer, diabetes, arthritis, etc. The advances have been mostly in the surgical arena and military medicine. Even with the great technological advances, they have not gotten closer to curing any of the major diseases. Heart disease has been the number one killer for over 80 years, yet we are not any closer to a cure.

According to an analysis that was published in the British Medical Journal, over 251,000 Americans die from medical errors each year. This is more than Alzheimer's, respiratory disease, strokes, accidents, and many more. Heart diseases and cancer are the only two conditions that claim more lives.

Many doctors tell us we can get all the nutrients we need from eating good quality food. That advice has harmed the health of millions and millions of people. While it is important to eat good quality food and avoid or at least limit junk and processed foods, no matter how good of a diet you have, you will not get all of the nutrients you need to be healthy. It is impossible. You will need to supplement to avoid becoming vitamin and mineral deficient and opening yourself up to many illnesses caused by nutrient deficiencies.

I have a lot of friends who are doctors, and I know these people went into medicine to help people and make a difference in people's lives. They have really good hearts. Unfortunately, in medical school, very little nutrition is taught. In all the time and years students spend in medical school, they will only spend from three to twenty-five hours total studying nutrition in classes. The message they get is that nutrition is not that important; otherwise, they would spend a lot more time studying nutrition. That is why many of them don't focus on nutrition but on treating with medical drugs, which is what they were taught in medical school.

Drugs don't cure. They only mask the symptoms. They don't treat the underlying cause, so you are not cured of anything.

According to the WHO (World Health Organization), the United States ranks only 69th in the world in the overall health of its citizens. Twenty-five years ago, we were 20th. What is going on? We are supposed to have the best healthcare in the world and spend the most money, yet we only rank 69th in the health of our citizens worldwide.

It is estimated that about 21% of all drugs prescribed by Medical Doctors are prescribed for what is called "off-label" use. This means that 21% of the time the doctor prescribes a drug for a disease or condition it has not been proven to treat.

Stephen Bruning, MD, headed the research on Ritalin during the 1970s and 1980s. He was caught cheating and charged with falsifying his research in 1988. Bruning was sentenced to 60 days in jail, fined $11,000, and received five years' probation. Yet, in an ironic twist, his fraudulent research helped stimulate the increased use of Ritalin both in the United States and abroad.

Did you know that 5 of the 14 medical experts who wrote the recommendations promoting the use of statin drugs to reduce LDL cholesterol and total cholesterol (using data from the "Framingham

Study") later admitted to having financial ties to the pharmaceutical companies that make statin drugs?

Did you know that there are studies that show men and women with cholesterol levels above 400 have fewer problems than those with low cholesterol levels?

Studies by the CDC from 1992-1995 show that 84%, 87%, and 76% of the flu people got were not in their shots. It was the wrong variant. Dr. J. Anthony Morris, former Chief Vaccine Control Officer at the FDA (Food and Drug Administration), said, "There is no evidence that any influenza vaccine thus far developed is effective in preventing or mitigating any attack of influenza. The producers of these vaccines know that they are worthless, but they sell them anyway."

Not only is it ineffective, but the flu shot sometimes causes damage. There is a correlation between the flu shot and Guillain-Barre' Syndrome. Because of many cases of Guillain-Barre' paralysis that occurred from taking the flu vaccines led to about 4,000 lawsuits. It resulted in over three billion dollars being paid out in compensation. I bet you never heard this from the makers of the flu vaccines.

The FDA states that only drugs can cure anything. If I come across an herb and discover that it cures some form of cancer and then try to sell it, that herb would be considered an illegal and unapproved drug, and I would get into big trouble.

Most directors of the FDA's medical research and drug departments are medical doctors with financial ties to the pharmaceutical companies.

The only prescribed drugs that cure anything are antibiotics, and there are a couple of problems with them. First, antibiotics kill both the bad bacteria and the good bacteria that your body needs. Our gut health and immune system suffer unless you replenish your gut with good bacteria. Second, as we use more and more antibiotics, many of the bugs have become resistant to them, and some of the antibiotics have become useless. Big Food often works with Big Pharma. The food industry paid off scientists in the 1960s to exonerate sugar and finger saturated fats as the bad guys, and that is one of the reasons there was a switch to a high-carb/low-fat diet that has wreaked havoc on people's health over the decades.

Big Pharma spends a lot of money advertising on television stations, and they make sure you don't see commercials stating the benefits of vitamins and minerals or news stories about how vitamins and minerals will help your health. You will often see bogus studies that state that a certain vitamin doesn't work or is dangerous to your health. Usually, these studies will either have a synthetic version of the vitamin (which you should not take) or a dosage that is really tiny or big enough to kill a horse. They don't mention that when they tell you the results of the study. Too much of anything will kill you. If you have too much water or too much oxygen, it can kill you.

For Big Pharma, a patient cured is a patient lost.

Here are the earnings of the Top 10 Pharmaceutical Companies in 2022:

1. Pfizer $100.33 Billion
2. Johnson and Johnson $94.94 Billion
3. Roche $66.26 Billion
4. Merck & Co. $59.28 Billion
5. AbbVie $58.05 Billion
6. Novartis $58.05 Billion
7. Bristol Myers Squibb $46.16 Billion
8. Sanofi $45.22 Billion
9. Zeneca $44.35 Billion
10. GSK $36.15 Billion

The global pharma market is expected to be $1.7 trillion by 2025.

Chapter 4
Why Wheat is Bad For You

Another villain a lot of people are not aware of is modern wheat. People are often told to eat wheat as it is good for them. The wheat that people eat today is much different from the wheat that was eaten for thousands of years. The current wheat is smaller and has a greater yield than the traditional wheat (e.g., einkorn). The problem is when they were setting up the current wheat, and they never bothered to do any animal or human safety testing on the new strains of wheat that were created. They just assumed there would be no problems with people eating the new wheat. They were dead wrong! Changes in traditional wheat were slow and gradual. In the mid-20th century, the genetic changes in wheat were massive, and the increase in yield went up tenfold. But this came at a price. Today's wheat and bread bear little resemblance to traditional wheat and traditional bread.

People who get off of modern wheat report being thinner, having better concentration, having fewer mood swings, thinking more clearly, having better joint and lung health, having more energy, and having better bowel movements.

Many people are not aware that when you eat wheat bread, your blood sugar skyrockets. It increases blood sugar as much as or even more than table sugar. Wheat is in so many products. You go to the supermarkets, and there are lots of products with wheat. Just read the labels and ingredients—breads, pasta, cookies, cereals, beer, frozen pizza, etc.

Gluten protein makes modern wheat doughy, spreadable, rollable, and stretchable. Because of gluten, a pizza maker can roll and toss the pizza dough and make it into the round, flattened shape we all know. About eighty percent of the protein in wheat is gluten.

The gluten in modern wheat has a much more harmful effect on health than that in traditional wheat, wreaking havoc on your intestinal lining by getting rid of the villi. There has also been a massive increase in celiac disease in the last 60 years, which correlates to when we started using modern wheat.

In case you thought that the gluten in wheat was bad, Dr. Robert Lustig writes in his book *Metabolical*, "Wheat also has seven hundred different proteins you could have an intolerance to - only two of them are the ones in gluten. The other 698 are just as capable of generating an immune reaction."

Eating wheat has also been linked to irritable bowel syndrome and acid reflux.

Ancient wheat has more protein than modern wheat and more other nutrients.

Dr. William Davis writes in his book *Wheat Belly*, "Aside from some extra fiber, eating two slices of whole wheat bread is really little different, and often worse, than drinking a can of sugar-sweetened soda or eating a sugary candy bar."

Dr. Davis also mentions that wheat products increase blood sugar levels more than just about any other carbohydrate. He explains, "This has important implications for body weight since glucose is unavoidably accompanied by insulin, the hormone that allows entry of glucose into the cells of the body, converting the glucose to fat. The higher the blood glucose after consumption of food, the greater the insulin level, the more fat is deposited." This goes contrary to all the advice you have been given that you should be eating lots of wheat and that it is good for your health. It is not healthy at all. As a result of what it does to blood sugar and insulin, modern wheat has been linked as a major cause of diabetes and obesity.

Wheat is also an appetite stimulant. It makes you want to eat more.

The truth is if you lose the wheat, you will eventually lose the belly. A lot of people try to go wheat-free and gluten-free. One warning about some of the gluten-free foods is that many of them replace wheat with tapioca starch, potato starch, corn starch, and rice starch. These foods will also greatly spike your blood sugar levels, so avoid gluten-free foods that contain these ingredients.

Wheat has also been linked to arthritis and pain in the joints. It is also linked to osteoporosis, especially in those with celiac disease.

Wheat also makes your body more acidic.

Wheat has also been linked to increased seizures in people.

Wheat consumption is the second leading cause of iron deficiency and anemia.

What can cause wrinkles, lost elasticity to the skin, and acne? Carbohydrates lead to acne, and wheat is a carbohydrate. Foods that increase blood sugar and insulin lead to the formation of acne.

If you are worried about not getting enough fiber in your diet, if you eliminate wheat from your diet, you can replace it with raw nuts and vegetables (and even some fruit), and your fiber intake will be fine. You can take psyllium husk fiber supplements (make sure they are organic) to help get enough fiber into your diet.

When you get rid of wheat, it will help improve the absorption of the various B vitamins, magnesium, zinc, and iron.

Chapter 5
Why You Should Avoid Vegetable and Seed Oils

Vegetable and Seed oils are foods you should stay away from and limit as much as possible in your diet.

Some types of vegetable oil include corn oil, cottonseed oil, soybean oil, safflower oil, peanut oil, and canola oil. Vegetable oils are made from seeds, nuts, grains, or parts of fruits. They are not natural. They have to go through a hydrogenation process, which makes them more harmful to your health.

Partially hydrogenated oils contain trans fats, which are very bad for you.

The FDA finally took the step of declaring PHOs (Partially hydrogenated oils), which were then the primary source of artificial trans fats in food, as no longer being GRAS ("Generally Recognized as Safe").

For most of the uses of PHO (Partially hydrogenated oils), June 18, 2018, was the date after which food companies could not add PHOs to foods.

The FDA decided to allow for a more orderly transition and extend the final date for compliance to January 1, 2021, to allow more time for products to work their way through distribution to not have PHOs.

Most of the inflammatory Omega 6's come from Vegetable Oils, which messes up the Omega 3/Omega 6 ratios.

Palm oil and coconut oil are safer and more stable, and they are not solid without having to go through the hydrogenation process like the other oils.

The Western diet has omega-6 LA consumption between 8 to 12% of total dietary consumption, which is much higher than the 2% that the traditional ancestral diet had. Linoleic Acid (LA) is an essential fat but is needed only in small quantities. Consuming large quantities of Linoleic Acid (LA) causes a toxic, pro-inflammatory, pro-oxidative, and nutrient-deficient biological environment. Linoleic acid is also extremely high in the current Western diet.

Vegetable or seed oils have risen to almost zero consumption in 1865 to nearly ⅓ of all the calories in the US and almost ¼ of all calories in 12 countries.

If you think that plant-based burgers are healthier than meat-based beef burgers, it turns out that plant-based burgers, on average, have almost six times the amount of linoleic acid than meat burgers (15.66% to 2.65%).

Cottonseed oil was primarily used for machine oil and lamp oil before 1865. Popular Science summed up an early 20th-century issue about cottonseed and cottonseed oil by stating, "What was garbage in 1860 (cottonseed), was fertilizer in 1870, cattle feed in 1880, and table food and many other things else in 1890."

Only 0.5% of the total caloric energy consumed as Linoleic Acid is considered essential. That is all you need.

Canola oil is repurposed engine oil. Fifty years ago you would have found it only in the shops of mechanics. Now canola oil is found in many foods. You don't want to be eating repurposed motor oil.

Vegetable oil consumption was about zero grams in 1865 and 1.62 grams per day in 1900. That jumped to 19 grams a day by 1960 and 80 grams a day by 2010.

Proctor and Gamble introduced the first trans fats on a very large scale using the brand name Crisco. Crisco was created to replace the more expensive pork lard and butter.

In 1961, the American Heart Association (AHA) recommended that men (and later women) reduce their saturated fat intake, stop eating butter, and replace it with vegetable oils to protect against heart disease. What the AHA did not tell people was that it had a conflict of interest. The AHA had accepted $1.8 million from Procter and Gamble (about $20 million in today's dollars) in 1948, and of course, P&G conveniently happened to make Crisco Oil. Procter and Gamble continue to support the AHA up to this day.

Conagra, Unilever, Mazola, Wesson, and other vegetable oil companies also got into the business of supporting nutrition researchers.

When you see organizations like the American Heart Association state that vegetable oils lower cholesterol, remember that they do so by oxidizing your lipoprotein particles, essentially burning them. This process can damage your arteries.

In 2015, the FDA announced that trans fats were removed from the GRAS (Generally Regarded As Safe) status, with extensions going up until January 2021 to remove trans fats from foods. The truth is that in 2024, there are still foods that contain trans fats. If you see anything that says "partially hydrogenated oils," that means there are still food manufacturers ignoring the FDA and putting trans fats in foods. As far as can be ascertained, no legal actions or penalties have been levied against these companies for putting trans fats in foods.

The FDA also allows American food manufacturers to label foods as having zero trans fats if they have less than 0.5 grams of trans fat per serving.

The average American eats about 80 grams of vegetable/seed oil daily, about 5.7 teaspoons. So if each serving of oil contained 0.49 grams of trans fat, the person could consume almost 3 grams of trans fat because the label says 0 grams of trans fat per serving. It should be noted that the FDA has stated there is no level of trans fat that is considered safe to consume.

During the 1980s, our diets became filled with seed oil, especially corn and soybean oil. Plus, corn was being fed to farm animals and fish, which increased the omega-6 consumption of their diet and ours. Human consumption of omega-6s tripled during the twentieth century. Linoleic acid concentration (the main omega-6 fatty acid) in our adipose tissue increased from 9 percent in 1959 to 21 percent in 2008. Omega-6 fatty acids are very pro-inflammatory and lead to a whole bunch of health issues.

Vegetable oils have none of the fat-soluble vitamins A, D, and K2, which are necessary for growth.

Rats that were given only vegetable oils as a source of fat showed stunted growth, got sicker, and died more quickly than rats given butter fat.

Seed oils have high levels of linoleic acid, which causes the LDL levels to become more susceptible to oxidation. Oxidized LDL has been shown to be a big factor in coronary heart disease and atherosclerosis (hardening of the arteries).

We only need 0.5% Linoleic Acid in our diet. The average Western diet has between 8 and 12% Linoleic Acid, which is 16 to 24 times what we need. Needless to say, such a high amount of LA in our diet makes us more susceptible to illnesses and diseases.

Vegetable/seed oils have been linked to cancer, heart disease, diabetes, obesity, age-related macular degeneration (AMD), and various other illnesses.

Dr. Chris Knobbe states in his book, *The Ancestral Diet Revolution*, "It is perhaps the fat-soluble vitamins A, D, and K which are the most important to us during all stages of life. The substitution of seed oils for animal fats, as we've reviewed, has substantially displaced the consumption of these fat-soluble vitamins, thereby leaving large percentages of populations undernourished and on the brink of depletion of these critical nutrients."

Consuming an excess of seed/vegetable oils creates a pro-inflammatory, pro-oxidative, nutrient-deficient, and toxic biological environment. This makes people more susceptible to massive weight gain and a whole bunch of chronic diseases.

It seems that excess Linoleic Acid and its breakdown products Advanced lipoxidation end-products (ALEs) play a major role in girls having their first period very early. Girls used to get their first period mid to late teens, and now many are getting it preteens and some as young as nine years old.

Nina Teicholz writes in her book, *The Big Fat Surprise Why Butter, Meat & Cheese Belong in a Healthy Diet*, "From the earliest clinical trials in the 1940s, in which diets high in polyunsaturated fats were found to raise mortality from cancer, to these more recent 'discoveries' that they contain highly toxic oxidation products, polyunsaturated oils have been problematic for health."

Teicholz continues, "The fact vegetable oils also create toxic oxidation products when heated and trigger inflammatory effects linked to heart disease, are, it seems, less important to mainstream nutritional experts, whose focus hasn't wavered from cholesterol. Most Americans don't realize that their nutritional advice is based on such a narrow set of health concerns, nor that large edible-oil companies have been contributing funds to their trusted, gilding institutions, such as the AHA, as well as to schools of medicine and public health."

Dr. Joseph Hibbeln from the National Institute of Health has studied and researched the effect of omega-6 oils on our health. According to Dr. Hibbeln, underconsumption of omega-3 and overconsumption of omega-6 fats led to increases in the following:

- Heart Disease
- Obesity
- Type 2 Diabetes
- Autoimmune Disease
- Rheumatoid Arthritis
- Metabolic Syndrome or Pre-Diabetes
- Irritable Bowel Syndrome
- Inflammatory Bowel Disease
- Asthma

- Cancer
- Psychiatric Disorders

Another problem with consuming high amounts of PUFA (Polyunsaturated Fatty Acids) is that PUFAs can have a harmful effect on both the thyroid and metabolic health since they inhibit the cell's ability to utilize active thyroid hormone. The body can convert the hormone T4 to active T3. In order to be able to increase energy production, our cells must also be able to access T3. PUFA's interfere with the cell's ability to use the active thyroid hormone T3. Vegetable oils increase tight junction permeability and wreak havoc on your gut as a result. Tight junctions are important in intestinal barrier function because they maintain selective permeability. PUFAs can expand the permeability of tight junctions. This can lead to Leaky Gut Syndrome, which you don't want.

The Sydney Diet Heart Study ran from 1966 to 1973 and studied 458 men who had suffered a heart attack. These men removed saturated fats from their diets and replaced them with linoleic acid from (soybean oil), which is pro-inflammatory. The men saw their LDL levels decrease, but their risk of heart attack went up 62 percent, as did their risk of dying (by 70 percent).

The Minnesota Coronary Study from 1968 to 1973 followed nine thousand patients at nursing homes and state mental hospitals. The patients had saturated fat removed from their meals and replaced with linoleic acid from corn oil. This study also showed results where LDL went down, but heart disease and atherosclerosis did not go down, and, in fact, death rates increased. The authors could not explain the findings, so they never published them. The data was put in the lead author's basement. It was discovered forty years later by his son, who was a cardiologist at the Mayo Clinic, who went on to publish the findings that lay hidden for four decades.

Dr. William Mercola, in his book *Fat for Fuel*, writes, "Refined oils are deadly for a wide variety of reasons: they throw your omega-6 to omega-3 ratio out of balance, they are highly susceptible to oxidation (which kicks off a storm of free radical damage within your mitochondria), they carry high levels of pesticides because most vegetable oils are extracted from genetically modified glyphosate-soaked plants, and they become even more volatile and harmful when they are subjected to heat."

Basically, you want to limit your vegetable/seed oil intake as much as possible.

Chapter 6
Why Processed Foods Are Not Healthy

One thing that has contributed to the increase of chronic diseases over the decades is the huge increase in processed foods. When food is processed, they usually take out the fiber. This started during the Depression in the 1930s. When they tried to take food throughout the country, the food became rancid and spoiled. They discovered they could make the food last longer if they removed the fiber. Food lasted longer, but we lost much of the fiber in the food, which is critical for our health. Because of the lack of fiber, the processed foods are more harmful now. The gut is starved while the liver is flooded.

In processed foods, they also take out potassium and put in more salt. Processed foods also strip the food of magnesium while usually keeping the calcium in. This upsets the calcium-to-magnesium ratio that is vital to good health.

Food processing increases the risk of heart disease, diabetes, and cancer.

Processed foods add a lot of sugar to preserve it. Food bought from your local bakery will last 2 to 3 days. Food bought in the supermarket will last up to 2 weeks because of the added sugars.

Dr. Robert Lustig says in his book *Metabolical*, "It's not what's in the food, it's what's been done to the food that matters." He is talking about food processing. He also recommends protecting the liver and feeding the gut. I think that is excellent advice. Good, high-quality real food will protect the liver and feed the gut, while processed and ultra-processed foods will do neither.

Food is actually inherently good. The problem happens when the food is processed; all kinds of bad things have been done. Poisons are often added to the food, which will stuff the liver. Also, antidotes are often removed, which will starve our gut. The gut is supposed to be full of good bacteria that eat the fiber that comes down and keep everything good. Processed food strips the fiber out, and the hungry bacteria will then start to eat the mucus barrier of the intestinal cells, which often leads to a leaky gut and inflammation.

Fruit juice is not healthy for you. In fact, fruit juices often have the same amount or slightly greater sugar than sodas. Plus, the juices have had the fiber taken out of them, so you lose the benefit of fiber by drinking orange juice or apple juice, for example.

Cooking such as corn oil, canola oil, soybean, or vegetable oil are extremely bad for your health.

If you are going to cook, I recommend using Avocado, Coconut Oil, or even Lard. Yes, lard is safe to cook with.

Ultra-processed food inhibits cellular growth. Ultra-processed food is estimated to account for about 73 percent of US food in the supply line. It is 52 percent cheaper than foods that are less processed.

Dr. Chris Knobble writes in his book, *The Ancestral Diet Revolution*, "In the French Nutrinet-Sante Cohort Study, which was a large prospective analysis lasting from 2009-2017, researchers found that for every 10% increase in ultra-processed foods in the diet, an associated 12% increase in overall cancer and an 11% increase in breast cancer occurred."

Processed foods can be mostly defined by the presence of four characteristics: refined flours, added sugars, seed oils, and trans fats. There are so-called mystery ingredients like artificial sweeteners and flavors that are created by food scientists who work for Big Food manufacturers, which you can add to the list. For every 10% of your diet that is ultra-processed food, the risk of death goes up 14%. Ultra-processed diet percentage for adults is over 60%, and for kids, it is 67%. That is very alarming.

Since the FDA removed trans fats from the Generally Regarded As Safe (GRAS) foods list in 2015, many people think there are no trans fats in foods anymore. Dr. Chris Knobbe writes in The Ancestral Diet Revolution, "However, trans fats exist within seed oils of many types and are not considered as being in violation of food policy by the U.S. F.D.A."

Chapter 7
Carbohydrates Are Not as Healthy as you May Think

People have been told for many decades to eat lots of carbohydrates. Sadly, for many years, people listened to their doctors who recommended they go on a low-fat/high-carbohydrate and egg-restricted diet. This led to an explosion of heart disease and heart attacks and increases in obesity and diabetes.

Carbs raise your blood sugar (fiber is an exception). Your net carbs are equal to the amount of total sugars minus the amount of fiber. While many people think that it is too much fat that makes you fat, it is too many carbs that lead to obesity. Farmers know this, so when they want to fatten up their animals, they feed them carbs such as grain and corn. They don't feed them fats.

The big killer is fructose. Glucose can be metabolized by various organs and is used by the cells as an energy source. Pretty much every cell can break down glucose into cells.

The same can't be said for fructose. Fructose can only be metabolized by the liver, and too much fructose can damage the liver. When too much fructose enters the liver, the liver uses excess fructose to create fat. This is done by a process called lipogenesis. If this keeps up and too much fat is stored in the liver cells because of the excess fructose, this can lead to a condition called non-alcoholic fatty liver. Millions of people have this non-alcoholic fatty liver and don't even know it.

The fructose in fruits is not as harmful because the fiber in the fruit partially offsets it, and it tells the brain that it is full.

NAFLD (Nonalcoholic Fatty Liver) is the leading cause of liver transplants in the United States. It was pretty much unheard of 45 years ago. Over a quarter of all teens (25%) now have fatty liver disease, which you only used to see in elderly alcoholics.

Fatty liver disease used to be caused by drinking lots of alcohol, which actually has a lot in common with fructose in its effects on the body. Now, forty percent of the adult population in the United States is affected by NAFLD, as well as a quarter of the world's population (25%). There are two stages of fatty liver disease. The first occurs when liver fat is deposited. The second stage is inflammation. Drinking lots of soda and other sweetened beverages with fructose can be damaging at both stages. The trans-fats in fried and highly processed foods are also harmful at both stages.

The occurrence of type 2 diabetes is about 20% greater in nations where high fructose corn syrup is easily available compared to those nations where it is not easily available.

Dr. David Perlmutter writes in his book *Drop Acid*, "Our dietary habits took a particularly devastating turn for the worse between 1970 and 1990, when the consumption of high-fructose corn syrup ballooned more than 1,000 percent - an increase that far exceeded the changes in intake of any other ingredient or food group. This has paralleled the rise in obesity and other conditions aggravated by high uric acid. Today, in the United States, dairy products, cereal grains (especially the refined form), refined sugars, refined vegetable oils, and alcohol make up a little more than 72 percent of the total energy consumed daily. These types of foods would have contributed little or no energy to the typical preagricultural hominid diet. In fact, the food industry that provides us with processed food has only been around for a scant 0.05 percent of the time that humans have been on this planet! We have not genetically adapted to thrive on our Western diet and lifestyles."

Eating food that will decrease your insulin burden by improving insulin sensitivity will lessen the burden of metabolic disease and allow the adipocytes to give up their stored fat. This will lead to weight loss.

Every day, the average American consumes 17 teaspoons (about 71 grams) of added sugar.

You may be surprised to find out that sweetness surpasses cocaine as a reward in rats. This tells you that sugar is very addictive, and many people are, in effect, sugar junkies. Coffee and soft drinks are price inelastic. When prices go up, sales don't go down much. The same is true for fast food.

Refine sugar, also called sucrose, is 50% fructose and 50% glucose. High fructose corn syrup is 55% fructose and 45% glucose. Sometimes, high fructose corn syrup has higher levels of fructose.

Sugar has been linked to cancer. Cancer cells feed off of sugar. Fructose is the worst.

Sugar prevents the absorption of Vitamin C into the cells.

Sugar increases blood pressure by increasing the amount of uric acid.

In 1960, 1 out of 100 people had Type 2 Diabetes. Today, it is about 1 out of 10. Many more children are getting diabetes.

More than twice as many people in the world go to bed obese as they do hungry, and not many people are talking about this very serious problem.

In 1960, 1 out of 7 people were obese. It is currently 1 out of 3, and by 2050, 1 out of every person in the US will be obese.

Almost 10% of kids have non-fatty liver disease.

Many people ignore the liquid calories from sugar-sweetened beverages like soda, juice, sports drinks, and sweetened coffees. These liquid calories are very dangerous because they go straight into fat production and storage. Plus, they are extremely addictive and increase your sugar cravings. Your body does not recognize these liquid calories as food, so you wind up consuming more total calories than if you had eaten solid food. These sweetened drinks have been known to cause obesity, heart disease, cancer, and type 2 diabetes.

Juices are bad because they are loaded with about the same amount of sugar as sodas, and unlike fruits, they are not offset in any way by fiber since fruit juices have pretty much no fiber in them.

Should you avoid carbs totally? No, I am not saying that. I recommend avoiding or at least limiting the sugars, fructose, and refined carbs.

You should eat plenty of fiber. Fiber does not raise blood sugar. People used to eat from millet but now use wheat and refined floor. Some say glucose is the sugar of energy utilization, while fructose is the sugar of energy storage.

Many doctors now believe that insulin resistance is the leading contributor to heart disease. Sugar poisons your mitochondria.

Food has a hormonal effect. Hormones control gaining and losing weight more than calories do. Carbs generally stimulate hormones that promote weight gain, while fat does not.

The military rejects lots of people because of obesity.

Kids today eat and consume far more sugar than they did decades ago.

Carnivores are generally not obese. You will never see a fat lion. Herbivores often are, such as the rhinoceros.

A study published in 2015 in the journal Circulation discovered that sugar-sweetened drinks kill 184,000 a year from obesity, cancer, and heart disease.

While fat works in your brain to curb your appetite so you will eat less during the day, sugar and carbs do the opposite. They will spike your insulin and promote fat storage. Sugar and carbs will also slow your metabolism and increase your cravings and hunger. And if you think that using artificial sweeteners, which you will find in diet sodas, is the way to go, guess again. They are known to cause type 2 diabetes, weight gain, alter your gut flora, increase hunger, and slow your metabolism. Yes, like sugars, artificial sweeteners can make you fat and diabetics. Yet, for some strange reason, the ADA (American Diabetes Association) recommends these artificial sweeteners, as do many diabetes doctors and even registered dieticians.

I am not saying to stay away from all carbs. Just stay away from the wrong carbs like processed foods, sugary cereals, refined grains, and snacks. Vegetables have carbs, but they are fine to eat. So go eat some green, leafy vegetables. Fiber is also a good carb and will not raise your glycemic index.

Chapter 8
Fats Are Healthier Than You Think

Fat has gotten a bad rap over the last 60 years, especially since many doctors told us that we need less fat and more carbohydrates, leading to the popular Low-Fat and High Carb Diets. If you eat a diet with plenty of fat and low amounts of carbs, you won't get obese.

Studies have found that those who eat fatty nuts have a lower risk of developing type 2 diabetes. Those who consume nuts daily and add a liter of olive oil a week have a significantly lower level of heart attacks and death.

The truth is fat does not make you fat. Carbs and seed oils make you fat. If you notice, carnivores don't get fat, while herbivores do. You will never see an obese lion, but you will see obese rhinoceroses. Lions also eat the fat parts of the animal they kill and the organ parts. They generally don't eat the lean part of the animal. Remember, when farmers want to fatten their animals, they give them carbs (grains and corn).

In his book *Eat Fat, Get Thin*, Dr. Mark Hyman writes, "In a recent review of fifty-three high-quality randomized, controlled trail that included 68,128 people and compared low-fat to high-fat diets lasting a year or more, the high-fat diets led to greater weight loss than the low-fat diets."

The Lyon Diet Heart Study, published in 1999, showed that a diet high in omega-3 fats lowered death from heart disease, cancer, stroke, and other diseases.

The Women's Health study was conducted over eight years and tracked 49,000 women. It showed that reducing fat in the diet did not prevent heart disease.

Lots of people have wondered why the French eat so much fat and butter, remain thin, and have lower rates of heart disease (the so-called French Paradox). Maybe we should be wondering why Americans eat less and less fat yet somehow keep getting fatter and fatter, as well as getting more heart disease. Perhaps the diet is a big factor in the difference between the French and the Americans.

Some of the benefits of dietary fats that many may find hard to believe include:

1. Dietary fats stimulate fat burning, lower your hunger pangs, and speed up your body's metabolism.
2. Dietary fat does not increase your overall calorie intake but reduces it.
3. Higher-fat diets promote weight loss more than high-carb diets. Plus, they are easier to stick to.
4. High-fat and low-carb diets can help reverse type 2 diabetes.
5. Dietary Saturated fat from coconut oil or butter does not raise the saturated fats in your blood.
6. The carbohydrates turn into saturated fats in your blood, which are the fats linked to heart disease.
7. Carbs turn on the production of fat in your liver. This is a process known as lipogenesis. This leads to high triglycerides and high cholesterol and lowers the good cholesterol (HDL). This also creates LDL particles that are small, dense, and heart disease-causing.
8. It's not fat that is responsible for the epidemics of obesity, type 2 diabetes, heart disease, and increased risk of dementia. It is refined carbs and sugar that are responsible.
9. Excess carbs slow your metabolism and stimulate your appetite and storage of belly fat.

Saturated fats are the least likely type that will oxidize. These fats don't cause heart disease and can protect us from heart disease. Eating dietary saturated fats does not raise blood saturated fats. Sugar and carbs (as well as excess protein) are what cause the liver to manufacture the saturated fats in your blood.

Saturated fats are vital fats that help provide structure and stiffness to your tissues and cell membranes. They help keep the cell's contents together. Eating a lot of omega-6 oils (e.g., vegetables, soy, or corn) will make our cells flimsy and floppy, and they won't function too well.

Trans fats are by far the worst fats and cause our cells to malfunction and create disease. Many foods and oils still contain trans fats.

Dr. Ronald Krauss, who used to chair the guidelines committee of the AHA (American Heart Association) during the 1990s, showed that saturated fat improves the so-called bad LDL cholesterol from the small, dense type that is dangerous to the type that is big, light fluffy, benign and safe LDL cholesterol. Carbs and sugar are most likely to lead to the small, dense, and dangerous type of LDL cholesterol.

One of the problems when people were told to switch to eating low-fat foods is that low-fat foods usually don't taste good. They had to improve the taste of the foods. What did they generally use to replace the fats? Yes, it was sugar. When you see so-called fat-free foods, check the ingredients. Usually, there is a ton of sugar in it, and the fat-free food will actually make you fat!

There is some good news on the fat front. In recent years, the American Cardiology Association and American Heart Association have abandoned the low-fat message and are not worried about dietary cholesterol. In fact, the Dietary Guidelines Committee in 2015 said, "Reducing total fat (replacing total fat with overall carbohydrates) does not lower CVD (cardiovascular disease) risk."

Dr. Rajiv Chowdhury, in 2014, reviewed 72 of the best studies on heart disease that covered over 600,000 people from over 18 countries. He came to the conclusion after reviewing the studies that saturated fat and total fat had no link with heart disease. The study also showed there was no support for the heavily promoted guidelines to increase polyunsaturated fats (e.g., vegetable oils). The study also found that omega 3 lowered heart disease while trans fats increased heart disease.

It turns out that the only time saturated fats cause inflammation is when there are high carbohydrate levels or low levels of omega-3 fats.

Saturated fats reduce inflammation when consumed with high fiber, high omega 3, and low carb diets. Inflammation is critical for both weight loss and healing.

Another study in Japan of over 60,000 people showed that eating more saturated fats actually led to a decreased risk of stroke.

If you triple your intake of saturated fats, it has no effect on the level of saturated fats in your blood. It is the carbs that raise your blood level of saturated fats.

Some benefits of saturated fats include:

1. They are vital for your nerves and nervous system to work well.

2. Saturated fats are necessary to make estrogen, testosterone, and other hormones.
3. Your lungs work better with saturated fats. Kids who get full-fat milk and better have lower rates of asthma than those who get margarine and low-fat milk.
4. Saturated fats help improve the immune system and make it strong
5. Helps brain health
6. Will help give you stronger bones.
7. Helps with liver health.
8. Saturated animal fats contain the important fat-soluble vitamins A, D, and K2 that are crucial for our health. Hunter-gathering diets had ten times the amount of these fat-soluble vitamins than the current average American.

Since saturated fat was replaced with refined carbohydrates in our diets, the rates of heart disease have increased.
Studies that have meat replaced by carbohydrates show the inflammation levels have increased.
Meat that is grass-fed raises levels of both omega-3s and the right omega-6s. It also aids in keeping the fats in balance. Large population studies show that people with the highest levels of omega-3s and arachidonic acid also had the lowest levels of heart disease and inflammation.
Restricting dietary carbs and vegetable oils and increasing fat will have the biggest impact on decreasing blood sugar levels.
As sugar, carbs, and seed oils consumption have increased, while fats have decreased, we have seen obesity and diabetes epidemics happen over the last 60 years.
It is also helpful to replace some carbs with proteins.
Dietary carbohydrates have a far bigger effect on saturated fat blood levels than dietary fats.
Low-fat diets have been linked with dementia and high fats have been shown to help prevent it and to treat it.
According to Dr. David Perlmutter, the author of *Grain Brain*, there is a lot of evidence to show that carbs bring about brain aging, and that fat helps prevent it.
A Mayo Clinic study discovered that people who eat lots of carbs quadruple their risk of getting pre-dementia. According to that same study, people who ate the healthiest fats had a 44 percent reduced risk of early dementia. Those who get quality protein from meat and

fish have a 21 percent decreased risk of early dementia.

You may know that your brain is 60 percent fat. Much of that comes from cholesterol and omega-3 fats. When a person eats a low-fat diet, he is starving his brain. Fat is very important for your brain. Lack of fat in the brain has been linked to mental disorders like depression and aggressive behavior, neurodegenerative disease, trauma, autism, ADD, and strokes. When people supplement their diets with omega-3 and other good fats, they see improvements in these conditions.

Bad fats like vegetable oils increase inflammation, while good fats lower inflammation.

High-fat, low-carb diets are anti-inflammatory and will decrease oxidative stress while you are exercising. They will also aid the body in recovering more quickly between exercise sessions and reduce lactic acid buildup.

Instead of worrying about getting too much fat in your diet, worry more about getting too much of the following: processed foods, carbohydrates (especially fructose), wheat, vegetables, and seed oils. They will wreak havoc on your health.

Chapter 9
Benefits of Fiber

I recommend that you get plenty of fiber, which is a carb that does not raise your blood sugar, as the body cannot digest and break down fiber. Most people are deficient in fiber and need more in their diets. You should ensure you get both the insoluble and soluble fiber in your diet.

Many people know that fiber helps you poop. While that is true, there is more fiber than just getting you to poop.

Research has shown that our ancient ancestors ate over 100 grams of fiber a day. Most people today, on average, only consume 15 grams of fiber a day.

Insoluble fiber adds bulk to the stool and is also called bulking fiber. It also helps food pass more rapidly through the intestines and stomach. Insoluble fiber will remain whole as it passes through the digestive system. This will help create a healthy stool and prevent constipation. It also speeds up the passing of waste through the gut. It does not absorb water or dissolve in water. Insoluble fiber can be found in brown rice, apples, pears, vegetables, beans, legumes, wheat bran, and potatoes.

Soluble fiber attracts water, can dissolve water, and turns to gel during the process of digestion. This helps slow down digestion. Soluble fiber is sometimes called viscous fiber. Soluble fiber is found in black beans, lima beans, oat bran, barley, nuts, seeds, avocados, and sweet potatoes. Soluble fiber can also be found in psyllium, which is a common fiber supplement. Fiber from veggies, especially green veggies, is also good, and I recommend eating them for your diet. Soluble fiber can stabilize blood sugar and decrease LDL cholesterol.

Fiber is not food for you. It is food for your bacteria. Fiber is an excellent prebiotic, which is food for good bacteria.

You also have prebiotics, which are called fermentable fibers. They help promote healthy gut bacteria as well as a healthy gut microbiome. According to various research, fermentable fiber may help prevent chronic inflammation. Preventing chronic inflammation may reduce various diseases such as heart disease, type 2 diabetes, and cancer. Foods containing fermentable fibers (prebiotics) include millet, asparagus, mushrooms, onions, artichokes, oatmeal, seaweed, lentils, bananas, and beans.

Many foods have combinations of different types of fiber. For example, avocados are about 80 percent insoluble fiber and 20 percent soluble fiber.

People used to eat millet but now use wheat and refined flour.

Fiber has several benefits. Here are some of them:

- Promotes regular bowel movement
- Support healthy hormone balance
- Gets rid of and binds with toxins
- Helps with the regulation of blood sugar
- Decreases fat absorption
- Gives you a feeling of being full or sated and reduces your appetite, which will bring about weight loss
- Supports healthy intestinal bacteria
- Boosts your intake of phytonutrients
- May lower the risk of heart disease
- Help your Gut Microbiome Thrive
- Can help prevent constipation
- Can help improve the mood

A high-fiber diet may help prevent certain forms of cancer, including colon cancer.

Fiber can also help with constipation.

Fiber slows down the release of blood sugar from the intestine to the bloodstream.

Fiber also helps with Inflammatory Bowel Disease (IBD) and Irritable Bowel Syndrome (IBS). Make sure to get enough fiber in your diet.

Fiber is also known to reduce the chronic inflammation and inflammatory process that frequently causes disease.

Women should get at least 25 to 28 grams of fiber per day. Men should get at least 31 to 34 grams per day. If that seems like too much, just remember our ancestors ate at least 100 grams of fiber a day.

Chapter 10
Why Getting Enough Sleep is Vital for Your Health

Sleep is very important and has so many benefits. Unfortunately, much of society and business look down upon people who sleep too much. And when I say look down on people who sleep too much, I mean 8 to 9 hours a day, not 16 hours a day. They tend to reward and idolize people who don't sleep. Companies like people who get little sleep and get to work early because they think they are better workers and get more done. The truth is that the more sleep you get, the more productive you are and the fewer mistakes you make.

Benefits of Getting Enough Sleep include:

- Gets rid of toxic proteins
- Promotes growth
- Helps with heart health
- Supports weight management
- Helps combat germs and keeps your immune system strong
- Reduces your risk of injury
- Increases attention span
- Boosts memory and learning
- Helps prevent infection
- Helps maintain a plentiful microbiome in your gut
- Can help prevent certain diseases

You may have noticed that often when you are sleep-deprived, you feel hungry. That is because when you sleep too little, there is an increase in a hormone that makes you feel hungry while at the same time suppressing a companion hormone that signals you are full and satisfied.

When you start having poor sleep, it triggers inflammation. Poor sleep will also impair glucose regulation and hormonal signaling. This leads to messing up your metabolism.

English scientists discovered in 2013 that being deprived of sleep for an entire week altered the function of 711 genes. Some of these genes include those dealing with inflammation, immunity, metabolism, and stress.

Many people are aware of all the deaths and accidents caused by drunk driving. Many people don't know that drowsy driving (e.g., falling asleep at the wheel) is a factor in 21% of fatal crashes.

It seems pretty much all of the organs in the body are enhanced by getting more sleep.

If you are a coffee drinker, you should be aware that caffeine has a half-life of 5 to 7 hours. That means it takes 5 to 7 hours to remove 50% of its concentration. If you have a cup of coffee around 7 pm, then at 1 am, you may still have 50% of the caffeine active and circulating throughout your brain tissue. This may be one reason you may have a bad night of sleep.

Sleep acts as a memory aid for both before and after learning. It helps your brain make new memories after learning, prevents forgetting, and cements those memories.

Athletes have a higher risk of injury if they consistently get less sleep.

NBA basketball players who get eight or more hours of sleep play more minutes, score more points per minute, show an increase in their 3-point shooting percentage, shoot better from the free throw line, have fewer turnovers, and commit fewer fouls than players who sleep less than 8 hours a day.

People who sleep less than 6 hours a day consistently make more mistakes and are less productive than those who get 8 hours of sleep daily.

Students who get 8 hours of sleep a day perform better at school on average than those who get 6 to 7 hours of sleep a day.

Much growth happens during sleep because, during the night, human growth hormone is secreted while we sleep. The National Sleep Foundation recommends that children between the ages of 6 and 13 get 9 to 11 hours of sleep, while teenagers between the ages of 14 and 17 get 8 to 10 hours of sleep.

Sleeping also allows your gut to repair itself.

Lack of sleep has been linked to behavioral problems, aggression, and bullying in children across various age ranges.

Over 60 percent of people with Alzheimer's have at least one clinical sleep disorder. One of the most common sleep disorders in Alzheimer's patients is insomnia.

A 2011 study linked progressively shorter sleep with a 45 percent increased risk of developing or dying from coronary heart disease within 7 to 25 years from the beginning of the study.

Another observational study in Japan of 4,000 male workers discovered an increase of 400 to 500 percent in suffering one or more cardiac arrests for those who sleep less than 6 hours a night than those who slept more than 6 hours.

People who sleep less tend to eat more and tend to have increased rates of diabetes.

Men who sleep too little or have poor quality sleep have a 29 percent lower sperm count than men who get a full and restful night of sleep. Men with less sleep also tend to have more sperm with deformities.

A European study of nearly 25,000 people concluded that sleeping 6 hours or less correlated to an increased risk of cancer of 40 percent compared to those who sleep 7 or more hours.

Dr. David Gozal at the University of Chicago did a study in which mice were injected with malignant cells, and he tracked the progression of tumors over the next 4 weeks. Fifty percent of the mice had their sleep partially disrupted, and the quality of their sleep was decreased and reduced. The other 50% were allowed to get enough sleep and sleep normally.

The sleep-deprived mice showed a 200 percent increase in the size and speed of the tumor growth compared to the well-rested mice group. When Dr. Gozal performed postmortems on the mice, he discovered that the sleep-deprived mice had far more aggressive tumors and their cancer had metastasized and spread to other areas of their body.

Ever notice that when you are trying to figure out a problem, when you get a good night's sleep, you often come up with an idea as to how to handle it the next day? That is one reason they say to sleep on a problem instead of staying awake on it. You are more likely to come up with that "Aha" moment after a good night's sleep.

A study by Dr. Ullrich Wagner at Lubeck, Germany, confirms this. The participants in his study were asked to work through hundreds of laborious numberstring problems. You can think of it like having to do a long division for an hour or two. The participants were not told that there was a shortcut they could use, which was common to all the problems. After the first session, where they worked on hundreds of these laborious problems, they were asked to return 12 hours later to work on more of these mind-numbing and laborious problems.

At the end of the second session, the researchers asked the participants whether they had figured out the shortcut rule to the problems. Some participants stayed awake for 12 hours, while others got 8 hours of sleep.

The group that got 8 hours of sleep had almost 60 percent get the "Aha" moment where they were able to figure out the shortcut or hidden rule. In contrast, only 20 percent of the group that stayed awake and tried to figure out a better way to solve the problems were able to figure out the shortcut common to all the problems. Other studies have shown similar results where the students figured out mazes and problems at a higher rate when they got 8 hours of sleep compared to those who got little or no sleep.

The blue light on computer screens affects your ability to sleep. You can either make sure to turn off your computer 1 to 2 hours before you go to sleep or you can lower the blue light on your computer screen in the evenings. Most computers and cell phones have this ability to lower blue light in the evenings.

You should also try to go to sleep around the same time each night, as your body will adjust to falling asleep at the same time each night.

Reducing or even eliminating caffeine and alcohol from your diet will help you sleep better. If you have to drink coffee, drink it early in the day.

Try not to exercise too close to bedtime, as exercising will likely keep you awake and alert, and you will have trouble falling asleep.

A century ago, only two percent of Americans slept less than 6 hours a day. Now, almost thirty percent get less than 6 hours of sleep a day. Trying to catch up on sleep on the weekends will not help much. You need to consistently get enough sleep every night.

Dr. Lewis Terman, a psychologist from Stanford who was also known for helping create the IQ Test, charted all the factors that aided the intellectual success of a child. Dr. Terman discovered that an important factor was getting enough sleep. In his book "Genetic Studies of Genius," Terman discovered that regardless of age, the more and longer a child slept, the more intellectually gifted the child became.

Dr. Ronald Wilson from the Louisville School of Medicine began a study in the 1980s that continues to this day. The research mainly focused on twins who, from a younger age, had one twin getting less sleep than the other and compared their developmental progress over the ensuing decades.

They discovered that by age 10, the twin who got more sleep had superior educational and intellectual abilities, had a greater vocabulary, and achieved higher scores on standardized tests of comprehension and reading than the twin who got less sleep.

The leading cause of death among teenagers is dying in traffic accidents, and very likely, a lack of sleep while driving is a big factor in this. Matthew Walker, PhD, in his book, *Why We Sleep: Unlocking the Power of Sleep and Dreams*, gives two examples of places where they changed the school start time to a later time and saw a big reduction in teen driving accidents.

In Teton County, Wyoming, they shifted the starting school time from 7:35 am to 8:55 a.m. The result was a 70 percent reduction in traffic accidents among those 16 to 18 years old. The Mahtomedi School District in Minnesota also pushed back the starting time of school from 7:30 am to 8:00 am. The result was a 60 percent reduction in traffic accidents among teenagers 16 to 18.

Hopefully, these facts show you why getting enough sleep each night is important. It has numerous benefits for you.

-

Chapter 11
The Importance of Having a Healthy Gut

The health of your gut is crucial to your overall health. Seventy percent of your immune system is in your gut. If your gut is not healthy, you won't be healthy. Dr. Josh Axe writes in his book *Eat Dirt: Why Leaky Gut May be The Root Cause of Your Health Problems and 5 Surprising Steps to Cure It*, "The gut is not simply a food-processing center - the gut is the center of health itself." Hippocrates, the Father of Modern Medicine, said, "All disease begins in the gut."

Your immune system is made from protein.

Your gut bacteria have a mind of their own and want to be fed. If you don't feed them, they can and will release neuroactive factors that can alter your behavior. And if you don't feed your good bacteria, the bad bacteria will multiply and send out inflammatory mediators that will cause inflammatory responses, leading to disease.

Probiotics are actually living bacteria. The intestinal environment has been made very inhospitable because of processed foods, antibiotics, seed oils, and sugars, and it's very difficult for good bacteria to live in that environment. Your gut needs to be fed, but processed food will starve it. This can lead to all kinds of health issues, such as metabolic syndrome, autoimmune disease, and intestinal issues.

There is a big connection between the gut and the brain.

One of the things that destroys gut health is antibiotics. While antibiotics kill the bad bacteria, they also kill the good and beneficial bacteria that are crucial to our health.

Another thing that destroys gut health is sugar. Processed foods are also bad for your gut. Fiber is eaten by the bacteria in our gut, which consider it food.

A healthy gut contributes to a strong immune system. A healthy gut also contributes to a better mood. Eighty to ninety percent of the serotonin is produced in the gut. It seems doctors have been looking at the wrong area for feeling good and depression for decades, as only 10% to 20% of serotonin is produced in the brain. Fifty percent of dopamine also comes from the gut.

Exercising regularly can also help protect your gut. Working out can increase the growth of healthy microbes in your gut. It can also increase the bacterial metabolite butyrate, which promotes gut barrier integrity and stimulates epithelial cell proliferation.

In her book, *Why Is America So Sick?*, Dr. Joanne Conaway talks about the importance of healthy bacteria in our gut. Dr. Conaway writes, "Healthy bacteria like the lactobacilli are responsible for several things:

- Better absorption of foods because of the enzymes they produce
- Increase in peristalsis wave of contraction that moves food through the intestine, helping to normalize bowel movements
- Increase in immunity through the secretion of acids and natural antibiotics
- Maintenance of good hormonal balance
- Vitamin production, especially the B vitamins
- Stabilization and balancing of cholesterol levels
- Defending against foodborne illness
- Keeping the intestinal walls fed by creating short-chain fatty acids."

There are lots of things that can destroy our gut health. They include antibiotics, sugars, prescription drugs, x-rays, processed foods, radiation, stress, antacids, gluten, chlorinated water, alcohol, tobacco, caffeine, and vegetable/seed oils.

If you don't take care of your gut, one of the results could be a leaky gut.

The gut microbiome is made up of all the various microorganisms that live in or on humans. They include all the various bacteria, viruses, fungi, parasites, yeast, and others).

We have a symbiotic relationship with trillions of microorganisms in our gut. The organisms have a mix of positive/good guys, negative/bad guys (e.g., pathogens), and neutral guys that go with the flow. The majority of experts believe that an average healthy microbe mix is 85 percent positive/neutral guys and 15 percent negative guys. This leads to a lively balance that leads your immune system to be alert and well-trained to defend against antigens and unhealthy viruses.

Bacteria outnumber human cells by a factor of ten to one. You actually have a hundred trillion bacteria in the intestines.

Leaky gut syndrome is also known as increased intestinal permeability. Leaky gut syndrome has been linked to many diseases, illnesses, and conditions such as ALS (Lou Gehrig's Disease), Alzheimer's Disease, Depression, Autism, Candida and yeast overgrowth, Celiac Disease, Type 1 and Type 2 Diabetes, Crohn's Disease, Chronic Fatigue Syndrome, Fibromyalgia, Gas and Bloating, Irritable Bowel Syndrome, Hashimoto's Disease, Metabolic Syndrome, Migraines, Multiple Sclerosis, Parkinson's Disease, Ulcerative Colitis, Allergies, Food Sensitivities, Rheumatoid Arthritis, Skin Inflammation (e.g., Acne, Psoriasis, Eczema, and Dermatitis).

We are 90 percent microbial on a cell-for-cell basis.

Studies have shown that increasing your fiber intake from fruits and vegetables will increase bacterial richness and help improve health issues. This is because you are feeding your good bacteria the fiber it needs.

Foods that can help protect your gut include bone broth, cooked vegetables, fermented dairy (e.g., kefir, cheese, and yogurt), fermented vegetables, natto, coconut products, and organic meats.

Stress (e.g., mental and emotional) can mess up our gut health and cause leaky gut syndrome. Stress can make you sick and worse pretty much every health condition out there. The gut-brain-microbiota axis allows the microbes and nerve cells in the gut to communicate with each other and with the brain. Thus, the gut and the brain affect each other. If you get stressed, it can affect your gut as well.

If you produce more stress hormones, you increase inflammation. More inflammation can irritate the lining of your stomach, which can lead to leaky gut syndrome or inflammatory bowel disease.

Make sure to lower your stress. You can do several things such as breathing deeply, exercising, taking a bath with Epsom salts or lavender oil, sitting quietly for at least 10 minutes a day, taking a break from your work and making time to socialize, and getting enough nutrition. Get enough rest. The great religions of the world have a sabbath to spend more time with God and have your body rest, so it does not break down from overworking.

Probiotics help restore the gut and also help with weight loss.

Prescription medications drain the body of many nutrients, which can lead to inflammation and leaky gut syndrome.

Probiotics will increase the levels of B vitamins, especially Vitamin B12, by improving the absorption of nutrients. And, of course, probiotics will improve leaky gut.

Chapter 12
The Awesome Health Benefits of Essential Fatty Acids (EFA's)

EFAs are also known as essential fatty acids.

EFA's consist of Omega 3's, Omega 6's, and Omega 9's. Omega 6's are important for your health. Very few people are deficient in Omega 6's. In fact, too much Omega 6's (the linoleic acid part) can be dangerous as it can lead to inflammation and many health issues.

EFAs help with balancing hormones. They help with sleeping. EFAs have been shown to lower triglycerides.

EFAs help with eyesight and heart disease. Short-term memory loss is often a sign of EFA deficiency. EFAs fight inflammation. EFAs also fight against cancer and Alzheimer's. EFAs help with blood pressure and with the baby's brain and eye development.

EFAs are required and necessary for the following processes:

- Proper adrenal and thyroid function
- Help with hormone production
- Development of cell membranes
- Regulation of blood pressure
- Help with heart health
- Aid in treating and preventing illnesses and diseases
- Regulating immune and inflammatory response
- Nourishing hair, skin and nails
- Aiding with breathing and lung problems
- Helping with brain health
- Aiding with liver function
- Breakdown and transport of cholesterol
- Proper growth and operation of both the nervous and brain system
- Aids in the regulation of blood clotting

Omega-3 EFAs oil reduces blood clotting, and Omega-6 EFAs stimulate blood clotting. You want to achieve a balance between the omega-3 and omega-6 fatty acids. Unfortunately, in most diets, there is an imbalance with a much higher rate of Omega-6 to Omega-3, which can cause health problems.

EFAs help boost vitamin and mineral absorption. EFAs promote proper functioning of nerves. EFAs also aid in normal growth and development.

Higher omega-3 blood levels were associated with an average increase in life expectancy of 4.7 years, according to a 2021 study. Another study discovered that having the highest omega-3 blood levels versus the lowest corresponded to a 34% lower risk of death.

Sources of Omega 3 fatty acids include:

- Flax Seeds
- Pumpkin Seeds
- Mackerel
- Salmon
- Cod Liver Oil
- Herring
- Sardines
- Soybeans
- Tofu
- Walnuts
- Dark Green Veggies like Collards, Chard, Parsley and Kale

Sources of Omega-6 fatty acids include:

- Nuts
- Tofu
- Almonds
- Seeds
- Kidney Beans
- Chickpeas
- Grains
- Legumes
- Dairy

The two main EFAs are omega-3 and omega-6. There is also omega-9. Omega-3s and omega-6s are essential, which means that your body can't make them. You have to get them from other sources. Since the body can make omega-9s from other fatty acids, they are not considered essential.

There are two types of unsaturated fatty acids: monounsaturated and polyunsaturated. EFAs are classified as polyunsaturated. They include:

- omega-3 fatty acid alpha-linolenic acid (ALA) and its derivatives, docosahexaenoic acid (DHA) eicosapentaenoic acid (EPA).
- the omega-6 fatty acid linoleic acid (LA), and its derivatives, arachidonic acid (AA) and gamma-linolenic acid (GLA).

These are the primary EFAs and their sources:

GLA (gamma-linolenic acid): The best sources of GLA include borage (starflower) oil (18-26%), evening primrose oil (7-10%), and black currant oil (15-19%). The typical diet supplies very little GLA.

LA (linoleic acid): can be found in most vegetable oils – safflower (55 to 77%), evening primrose seed (60 to 80%), sunflower (55-75%), corn (59%), peanut (33%), canola (20-26%), and olive (10%). LA is very abundant in the food supply. You don't need to supplement. The truth is you only need a tiny amount of LA, and most people have excessive LA levels, making them more prone to illnesses and diseases.

AA (arachidonic acid): Good sources of AA (arachidonic acid) are meat, fish, and eggs. AA is fairly abundant in the food supply. It can be found in all of your cell membranes and helps your body control inflammation, grow, and repair.

EPA and DHA: EPA (eicosapentaenoic acid) and DHA (docosahexaenoic acid) are found in fish like sea bass, oysters, sardines, shrimp, salmon, mackerel and tuna. Fish oil supplements contain 12-20% DHA and 18-30% EPA. They can also be found in krill oil and cod liver oil. Algal sources of EPA and DHA are also available.

ALA: ALA (alpha-linolenic acid) can be found in flax seeds (17-23%) and flaxseed oil (50-60%) and in chia seeds, walnuts, avocados, green soybeans, green leafy vegetables, oysters, canola, navy beans, wheat germ, and black currant seeds.

Diseases and disorders such as eczema, Premenstrual Syndrome (PMS), high blood pressure, diabetes, and rheumatoid arthritis have been linked to deficiencies in EFAs. Adding EFAs to your diet may help improve these conditions.

Diets abundant in ALA, DHA, and EPA aid in maintaining a healthy heart and might protect you against cardiovascular disease.

Because of the convincing and compelling evidence for EFAs

helping with heart health, the AHA (American Heart Association) in October 2000, the American Heart Association changed its dietary guidelines to recommend eating at least two servings of fish (especially fatty fish) per week.

Arthritis and other joint conditions

GLA (gamma-linolenic acid) is converted to eicosanoids, which fight inflammation. GLA also regulates the immune response, which can reduce inflammation of the joints. It turns out that many sufferers of rheumatoid arthritis have a deficiency in GLA (gamma-linolenic acid), react well when treated with GLA, and have shown reduced symptoms in placebo-controlled studies. People who were given GLA have experienced lessening of pain, joint swelling, and extent of morning stiffness. Another great thing with GLA supplementation is the decreased use of corticosteroids, antibiotics, and non-steroidal anti-inflammatory drugs (NSAIDs).

Eczema and other skin disorders have been linked to EFA deficiencies, especially GLA (gamma-linolenic acid). EFAs help relieve dry and itchy skin. I used to get dry skin every winter and would put hand lotions on it. Since I added EFAs to my diet, I haven't had dry skin issues on my hands during the winter in years. Over 22 randomized, placebo-controlled trials have been done with EFAs and eczema, with most of the trials demonstrating great benefit.

Omega-3s help with the brain, which is why they have been added to baby formula. Breast milk usually has lots of them as long as the mom has been eating them.

Omega-3 EFAs are also known for helping play a role in mental health.

EFA deficiencies have been linked to the following:

- Dementia
- Alzheimer's
- Bipolar Disorder
- Depression
- Attention Deficit Disorder
- Dyslexia
- Cognitive Impairment

Recent research dsuemonstrates that DHA and EPA may be helpful in treating depression as well as other mental illnesses according to recent research.

Some preliminary recent human clinical trials have been done in the area of cancer that are pretty encouraging. GLA (gamma-linolenic acid) has shown anticancer outcomes, both by itself and in cancer drugs like tamoxifen.

Consuming more Omega 3 can help lessen joint inflammation. EFAs are very important for your health. Make sure you are getting enough of it.

An imbalance between omega 6 and omega 3, where the omega 6 ratio is much higher to omega 3, causes all kinds of health issues. The higher ratio can lead to depressed immune system functioning, inflammation, and weight gain. When omega-6 levels get very high, it oxidizes your LDL cholesterol (the so-called bad cholesterol), making it more rancid and more likely to cause cardiovascular disease. Your blood also becomes more sticky and more likely to clot.

Chapter 13
Cholesterol is Actually Good For You?

Cholesterol is something you hear about all the time. You keep hearing that you have to lower your cholesterol; otherwise, you are susceptible to heart attacks and heart disease. They tell you to avoid eggs because eggs are high in cholesterol.

There is no correlation between cholesterol and clogged arteries. Cholesterol is important to the human body for many reasons:

1. All of your sex hormones are made of cholesterol.
2. Your stress hormones are made from cholesterol.
3. All of the insulation that wraps around your body's nerves are made from cholesterol.
4. All of the walls of the trillions of cells in your body are made from cholesterol.
5. Your brain is 2% of your body's weight yet has 20 to 25% of your body's cholesterol. About 60% of the brain's weight is fat, so you need plenty of cholesterol for optimal function.
6. Cholesterol does not cause heart disease.
7. Vitamin D is made from cholesterol.
8. Steroid hormones would not exist without cholesterol.
9. We would not have bile acids without cholesterol.

Your brain has a lot of cholesterol, and about 25 percent of the cholesterol resides in the brain. That should give you an idea as to how important cholesterol is. The fatty myelin sheath surrounding every nerve cell and fiber is about 20 percent cholesterol. Communication between neurons relies on cholesterol. There is a connection between mental function and naturally occurring cholesterol.

Cholesterol also plays an important role in helping fight infections and bacteria. A 15-year study of 100,000 healthy individuals in San Francisco discovered that the participants who had low cholesterol levels were far more likely to be admitted to the hospital with an infectious disease.

People who go on statin drugs lose their strength, energy, and appetite, and they often return after they go off of statin drugs. Statin drugs not only lower cholesterol in the blood but also lower it in the brain. That's not good news because your brain depends on cholesterol to function at its best. The brain may make up only 2 percent of the body, but it has 25 percent of the body's cholesterol.

Cholesterol is a crucial part of the brain's cell membranes. It also plays a vital role in neurotransmitter transmission. If you don't have cholesterol, communication between cells is damaged, brain cells won't be able to talk to one another effectively, and memory and cognition are adversely affected. People who are on statins for a long time tend to have more memory and cognition problems, and not surprisingly, there has been a huge increase in dementia and Alzheimer's disease as a result of statins and other cholesterol-lowering drugs.

We need cholesterol for bile acid production, and statins alter the composition and size of the bile acid pool. Bile acids play an important role in shaping the gut microbiome, so statins also affect the gut microbiome. They have been shown to reduce the diversity of gut bacteria (which leaves you more open to disease) and reduce the level of butyrate (which plays an important role in protecting against colon cancer).

Statin drugs are anti-inflammatory, which is probably one of the main reasons they show any of the benefits they occasionally do. Sexual dysfunction, particularly in men, could be related to the drug they are taking to lower cholesterol. Not only does the brain need cholesterol to function properly, but the gonads also require cholesterol to produce the hormonal fuel required to keep the sex life going for couples. The major sex hormones like estrogen, testosterone, and progesterone come from cholesterol. If you lower your cholesterol, you will lower your sexual function. Various studies have shown that taking statin drugs leads to a reduction in sex hormones, especially testosterone. Remember, in addition to men, women also have some testosterone (less of it, of course, than men), but even this small amount in women influences their sexual desire. In fact, the majority of anti-aging clinics prescribe tiny doses of testosterone to postmenopausal women who have low levels of sexual libido. Another study showed that the popular statin drug Crestor increased the risk of erectile dysfunction from two and up to seven times!

Low levels of testosterone are also linked to a reduced life expectancy as well as an elevated risk of mortality from cardiovascular disease.

Statin drugs may be linked with increased risk for both diabetes and cancer. One of the ways statin drugs promote cancer is by reducing the natural killer cell cytotoxicity. This reduces the body's immune response to tumor cells. Statins also increase the functionality and number of regulatory T-cells. This can weaken the body's immune system against tumors and lessen the effectiveness of immunotherapy in cancer treatment.

As for diabetes, a 2014 study was published in the journal Diabetes Care of 115,000 Italian residents who were treated with statins in 2003 and 2004 and followed for seven years. The more consistently the patients took their statin drugs, the higher the risk of developing diabetes grew. According to the researchers, "In a real-world setting, the risk of new onset diabetes rises as adherence with statin therapy increases." The people who consistently took the statin drug had a 32 percent greater risk of becoming diabetic compared to those who had a low adherence to taking the statin drug.

According to the ALLHAT study that lasted from 1994 to 2002, there was ultimately no difference in deaths between the group that took the statin drugs and the group that took no statins.

Lowering LDL does not reduce plaque.

Before stating drugs became popular in the 1990s, there were a bunch of studies in which various other drugs lowered cholesterol. One of them, known as fibrates, was the go-to treatment for cholesterol before statin drugs took over.

In the late 1980s, Russel Smith wrote the most comprehensive and critical review of diet-heart disease. It was published in two volumes that were over 600 pages and contained over 3,000 references. It was titled *Diet, Blood Cholesterol, and Coronary Heart Disease: A Critical Review of the Literature*.

Smith discovered that in the vast majority of studies he reviewed, there was no difference in the number of people who died between the group that did not lower its cholesterol and the group that did.

Dr. Edward Pickney wrote a book called *The Cholesterol Conspiracy*, in which he reviewed all the various diet-heart disease studies. Dr. Pickney found that the drugs lowering cholesterol were good at lowering cholesterol but not very good for anything else, e.g., saving lives.

The primary cause of heart attacks is not cholesterol but insulin resistance.

Eating foods high in cholesterol has little effect on your blood's cholesterol. So feel free to eat those eggs.

About 60 years ago, Dr. Ancel Keys became a proponent of what later became known as the lipid hypothesis. He concluded that too much cholesterol causes heart disease. He came to believe that saturated fat raises cholesterol levels. This became the basis of the lipid hypothesis: Saturated fats increase cholesterol levels, and high cholesterol levels (particularly LDL) cause heart diseases. In fact, whenever you hear about saturated fat, you often hear it referred to as "artery clogging saturated fat." It has never been proven true, so it is still called the lipid hypothesis. For the last 60 years, researchers have looked to prove the lipid hypothesis true, but they have not had much luck.

You have HDL (high-density lipoprotein), which many call good cholesterol. You also have the LDL (low-density lipoprotein), which many call the bad cholesterol. A type of lipoprotein with a small, dense LDL (aka type B LDL) may cause heart disease. The small and dense LDL particles are the ones that seem to cause or worsen atherosclerosis and increase plaque in the arteries. The low-fat high carbohydrate diet makes the type B LDL cholesterol worse. Guess what lowers the small, dense LDL particles? It is fat, especially saturated fat, that reduces the amount of small and dense LDL particles. High-fat and low-carb diets lower triglycerides, raise HDL cholesterol, and increase the harmless big and fluffy LDL particles—all of these lower the risk of heart attack.

According to Dr. Stephen Sinatra and Dr. Jonny Bowden in the book *The Great Cholesterol Myth*, "It turns out many people with 'high LDL' actually have a very low risk for heart disease. Conversely, many people with 'low LDL' can have a very high risk for a cardiovascular event. (This was true for one of the authors.)"

LDL is usually not a problem until it gets oxidized. That is because oxidized (that is, damaged) LDL can go under the arterial walls and begin the inflammatory process that eventually leads to the plaque being created. This leads to further injury and inflammation. Non-oxidized LDL is relatively harmless and travels through the mindstream without causing damage.

The big problem is the triglycerides, not the cholesterol. Sugars, processed foods, and starch will raise the triglycerides.

Dietary fats make only a small contribution to the production of VLDL (Very Low-Density Lipoprotein). Carbohydrates contribute a much bigger portion to VLDL. This is one reason low-fat diets high in carbs and so-called healthy whole grains increase triglyceride levels. In fact, low fat diets often send triglyceride levels from 150 mg/dl to 300 mg/dl range.

Foods that raise blood sugar levels the most also increase insulin the most. This leads to stimulation of de novo lipogenesis in the liver and a greater deposit of visceral fat in the liver. This will be followed by increased small LDL and VLDL (low-density lipoprotein)/triglycerides.

In their book, Sinatra and Bowden also state, "The real tragedy is that by putting all of our attention on cholesterol, we've virtually ignored the real cause of heart disease: inflammation, oxidation, sugar, and distress."

It turns out almost 70 percent of people who wind up in the hospital because of a heart attack have normal cholesterol levels.

The Nurses' Health Study discovered that 82 percent of coronary events could be attributed to five factors. None of those five factors was cholesterol.

The National Cholesterol Education Program lowered what they said were the optimal cholesterol levels in 2004. Eight of the nine people on the panel who made the recommendation had financial ties to the pharmaceutical industry.

The ENHANCED study trial for the cholesterol-lowering medication Vytorin waited two years after the study was completed (2006 to 2008) before releasing the results. The people taking Vytorin saw their cholesterol go down sharply. Great news, right? Unfortunately, it turns out the participants also had more plaque growth than those who took the standard cholesterol drug. Those who take Vytorin showed almost twice as much an increase in the thickness of their arterial walls, which is probably why they waited two years to release the results.

Numerous studies have shown that lowering the risk for heart disease has little correlation with lower cholesterol. Far bigger factors that initiate damage to the arteries include oxidation and inflammation.

For most of the population (over 95 percent), cholesterol in the diet pretty much has no effect on cholesterol in the blood.

The low-fat, high-carbohydrate diet will increase their number. High carbohydrate diets will not only raise triglycerides and lower your HDL but also make the LDL small and dense. All of this leads to an increase in heart disease.

There is also another type of LDL cholesterol that is large, fluffy, harmless, and beneficial. The LDL cholesterol drugs lower this type of LDL cholesterol.

In a study of almost 140,000 patients who went to the hospital for heart attacks and heart disease, about half had optimal LDL (bad cholesterol) levels of under 100 mg/dL. Yet many proponents of the lipid hypothesis, instead of rethinking their hypothesis, stated that even 100 mg/dL for LDL cholesterol is too high and needs to be reduced.

Did you know that our body considers cholesterol so important that the liver makes about 1,000 mg of cholesterol each day? The liver makes up 80% of the cholesterol. The kind of food you eat has little effect on your cholesterol. Your body knows what to do with cholesterol and will regulate and sort the cholesterol levels. If you are eating too much cholesterol, it will compensate by making less cholesterol. If you are eating too little cholesterol, your body will produce more cholesterol.

Much of your brain is made of cholesterol. There are a lot of great benefits to cholesterol.

Your body does a good job of keeping your cholesterol in check. If you eat foods high in cholesterol, your body will offset it by making less cholesterol in the liver. So if you eat several eggs at a meal, your body will compensate by making less cholesterol.

The latest science shows that when people's cholesterol levels are low, their brains do not function as well and function sub optimally. They are also at greater risk for dementia, depression, and other neurological problems.

Say you replace the saturated fat you eat with carbohydrates. Maybe instead of eating bacon and eggs for breakfast, you start eating cereal with skim milk and grapes or bananas. You may see your LDL go down. However, you will also see your triglycerides go up, and the triglycerides are the big problem.

Low HDL is also a factor for cardiovascular disease. You are much more at risk for having a heart attack if you have low HDL cholesterol than if your total cholesterol or LDL cholesterol is elevated.

You lower your HDL levels when you replace your fat (including saturated fat) with carbs. That means you raise your risk of a heart attack. So stick with eggs and bacon instead of cereal with skim milk and grapes.

The New England Journal of Medicine stated that HDL is a biomarker for dietary carbohydrates. In layperson's terms, if your HDL levels are high, you probably eat little carbs. If your HDL levels are low, you are probably eating a lot of carbs.

Years ago, you could find lard in every supermarket. Now, it's very difficult to find lard in most stores. Bakeries and fast-food restaurants used to use lard in great quantities. Later on, these places were pressured to replace lard with artificial trans fats that have wreaked havoc on people's health. They were pressured because they thought lard was a factor in heart disease. That has been shown to be false. Nearly half the fat in lard (about 47 percent) is considered good by just about everyone. That good fat is monounsaturated fat. Monounsaturated raises HDL cholesterol and lowers LDL cholesterol.

Olive oil, which is the darling of those who tout the Mediterranean diet, is 71% oleic acid, which is the monounsaturated fat that is good for the heart. Lard is about 44% oleic acid, which is more than sesame (41%), corn oil (28%), and cottonseed oil (19%).

If you replace the carbs in your diet with an equal amount of lard, you will lower your risk of getting a heart attack.

Without cholesterol, your bones would turn to slush because you would not be able to get vitamin D from sunlight. You also would not be able to absorb calcium.

Cholesterol is required for your sex hormones. Without cholesterol, we would not be able to engage in sexual intercourse, would not be able to procreate, and the human race would eventually become extinct. Sex hormones and stress hormones are made from cholesterol. Cholesterol is required to create cell membranes and coat nerves with a protective insulation of fat that comprises 60 to 80 percent of our brain tissue.

You also need cholesterol for fat absorption because it produces bile salts. Cholesterol is crucial for proper digestion of food.

The Inuit have cholesterol levels between 300 and 500 and have very little heart disease.

The acceptable level of high cholesterol keeps changing and keeps being lowered. A cholesterol level of 300 used to be acceptable, but then they kept lowering it several times until now, when the acceptable cholesterol level is 200.

If there is a measure that is a good predictor of both heart disease and insulin resistance, it is the ratio of your triglycerides to HDL. It will predict your risk of heart disease and insulin resistance. The higher the ratio, the greater your risk of heart disease. Ideally, you want the ratio to be about 2 to 1 (Triglycerides divided by HDL). If your ratio is 5, the risk of cardiovascular issues increases significantly. According to a Harvard study published in Circulation, a journal that the American Heart Association publishes, the people with the highest triglyceride to HDL ratios had an incredible 16 times the risk of developing heart compared to those with the lowest ratios.

It is not the cholesterol that causes heart attacks. It is the triglycerides. However, pharmaceutical companies have never been able to create a drug that lowers triglycerides. Nevertheless, they do have drugs that lower cholesterol called statin drugs. Thus, they have doctors focus on lowering cholesterol levels.

Statins have numerous side effects. They have been linked to dementia, Alzheimer's disease, memory loss and paranoia. They also increase your risk of diabetes. Statins can damage the liver and can cause headaches and diseases. They can also cause muscle aches and pains. Statins can also cause digestive problems, constipation, and sleep problems. They are also known to cause joint and abdominal pain. Statins have been known to damage the nerves and lower your levels of COQ10. Statins also help men more than women. On average, statins raise life expectancy by about four days. Is it worth experiencing all those horrible side effects so that you can live an extra four days? Maybe they should just focus on oxidized cholesterol instead of saying all cholesterol is bad.

A normal by-product of protein digestion is homocysteine. Homocysteine can build in your body if you don't have enough magnesium and B vitamins. Very high amounts of homocysteine can lead to oxidized cholesterol. Blood vessels are damaged by oxidized cholesterol.

Cholesterol makes your prostate happy and is responsible for 95% of the weight of your testosterone.

Dr. Joel Wallach writes in his book *Epigenetics*, "Alzheimer's disease is a physician-caused disease, produced by lowering cholesterol and saturated fats in the patient's diet, prescription of statin drugs, and the directive to avoid vitamin and mineral supplements. In fact, Alzheimer's disease is a physician-caused disease. Prevention of Alzheimer's has been documented by a Johns Hopkins randomized and double-blind study on almost 5,000 people over the age of 65. The ten-year study published in 2004 demonstrated clearly that the consumption of a special diet, avoidance of certain foods, and the supplementation of nutrients can reduce the risk of Alzheimer's disease by 78%. In April 2012, the FDA sent out an urgent warning, "Statin drugs increase the risk of dementia and type 2 diabetes!"

Chapter 14
Why Collagen is Crucial for Your Health

Collagen is the primary structural protein located in your body's various connective tissues. Collagen is the main component of connective tissue and the most abundant protein in humans and other mammals. It makes up from 25% to 35% of the entire protein content of the body. Collagen is primarily found in connective tissue such as ligaments, tendons, cartilage, bones, and skin. It comprises amino acids that are bound together and form a triple helix of extended fibril known as a collagen helix.

Throughout history, people have obtained collagen by eating real bone broth, and nearly every part of the animal has it.

Collagen makes up about 30% of your body's proteins. It is the most abundant protein in your body. Collagen is also the main protein in the connective tissue.

Collagen is found in your blood vessels, organs, and intestinal lining. It is also the primary building block of your body's bones, muscles, skin, ligaments, tendons, and other connective tissue.

Amino acids are what proteins are made of. Proline, glycine, and hydroxyproline are the main amino acids that make collagen. These three amino acids combine to make protein fibrils in a triple helix structure. The proper amounts of vitamin C, copper, manganese, and zinc are required to make the triple helix.

Vitamin E aids in the production of collagen.

The term collagen is derived from the Greek word "kolla," which means "glue," and the suffix "-gen," which means "producing."

Twenty-eight types of collagen have been identified so far.

- Type I. This type is the most abundant, making up 90% of your body's collagen. Type I is densely packed and used to provide structure to your skin, bones, ligaments, tendons, teeth, and the disk between the vertebrae. Taking Type I collagen will help promote skin health, wound healing, digestive health and lean muscle mass.
- Type II. This type of collagen can be found in elastic cartilage, which provides joint support. The highest concentration of Type II comes from chicken collagen. Type II will help safeguard joint health by providing flexibility and support for joints and helps with joint pain. It also supports the respiratory system and the organs.

- Type III. This type is found in the organs, blood vessels, muscles, and arteries. Type III collagen is often found together with Type I collagen.
- Type IV. This type of collagen is found in the layers of your skin.
- Type V. This type is found in the cornea of your eyes, liver, lungs, muscles, bones, some layers of skin, hair, as well as tissue of the placenta in pregnant women.
- Type X. This type of collagen aids in supporting cartilage maintenance and helps promote bone strength.

As you get older, your body makes less collagen, and the existing collagen breaks down at a quicker rate. Normally, people start losing collagen around the age of 25, and they lose a little collagen each year. As you age, the quality of the collagen is also lower than when you were younger. After menopause, women undergo a considerable reduction in collagen production.

Collagen peptides are small, fragmented pieces of animal collagen that are easily digestible. There is no vegetable collagen. Collagen cannot be absorbed in a whole form. Collagen must be broken down into shorter peptides or amino acids. The peptides are absorbed through your gastrointestinal tract. Collagen supplements can be in either powder or pill form. These supplements often contain two or three amino acids. The supplements are sold as either collagen peptides or hydrolyzed collagen. The peptides are broken down through a process called hydrolysis. When collagen is hydrolyzed, it becomes more bioavailable. In other words, it is more effectively absorbed by the body and is easy to digest.

Bone is a living and growing tissue. Bone is mostly made of collagen and is continuously being broken down and renewed. Collagen supports the bone-building process by encouraging stem cells to convert into bone cells and multiply.

Over 99 percent of the calcium in the body is contained in the teeth and the bones. The combination of calcium and collagen supports bone integrity and bone strength.

There are a whole bunch of health benefits of collagen.

Collagen does these things:

Collagen strengthens and improves your hair, skin, and teeth. Reduction in wrinkles, reduces skin stretch marks, and cellulite can all be the result of lower collagen. Your skin looks smoother and firmer the more collagen you eat.

It helps fix leaky gut

When a person gets a leaky gut, toxins can pass through the digestive tract and go into the rest of the body. When this happens, the toxins can wreak all kinds of havoc and damage the entire system. Collagen has been shown to help seal your intestines and repair a leaky gut. Collagen can help your digestion if you suffer from inflammatory bowel disease.

Collagen has anti-inflammatory properties and helps with treating pain. Collagen helps ligaments, tendons, and joints glide smoothly, similar to the oil in a car engine. Swollen, stiff, and painful joints are often the result of reduced collagen levels. Collagen has been shown to help alleviate osteoarthritis pain.

The amino acid glycine, found in collagen, is known to help convert glucose into energy, increase your metabolism and lean muscle. When you have more lean muscle, that translates to a faster metabolism because muscle burns off more calories than fat. This process is helped by taking vitamin C along with collagen.

Glycine aids in protecting the liver from toxins. Glycine can also help fix any liver damage.

Good for your heart and cardiovascular health:

The amino acid proline, which is also found in collagen, may help clear deposits of fat from arteries as well as help repair arteries. Proline also helps reduce blood pressure.

Food Sources of Collagen include:

- Bone Broth
- Fish
- Chicken
- Beef
- Gelatin
- Eggs
- Dairy
- Legumes
- Citrus Fruits
- Leafy Greens
- Berries

Signs of Collagen Deficiency include:

- Joint and Arthritis Pain

- Wrinkles and sagging skin
- Brittle Nails
- Weaker and smaller muscles
- Thin or dull hair
- Reduced bone density
- Immune problems
- Greater sensitivity to foods
- Cardiovascular Issues
- Gastrointestinal issues
- Constant cuts and abrasions
- Poor Wound Healing
- Blood Flow Issues
- Decreased mobility
- Fatigue
- Muscle Aches

Glycine interacts with cysteine and glutamine to manufacture glutathione. Glycine aids with synthesizing creatine. Creatine is important for building muscle, muscle recovery, energy output, and athletic performance.

Glycine can help you achieve more sleep. Taking 3 to 5 grams of glycine can give you restful and peaceful sleep. Glycine has been shown to impede the deterioration of muscle protein.

Arginine increases growth hormone levels, and that contributes to muscle growth.

Make sure you are getting enough collagen, especially as you get older.

Chapter 15
Salt is Actually Good for You

Salt is an essential mineral and nutrient that our bodies require to live. Salt has been vilified as something where too much of it is harmful to your health. The truth is that in most cases, more salt is better for your health than less. Most of the time, the negative health effects that many blame salt for result from sugar consumption.

In 1977, the government's Dietary Goals for the United States recommended that Americans restrict salt intake. A report from the U.S. Surgeon General released around the same time as the Dietary Goals admitted that they could find no evidence that eating a low-salt diet would help prevent the increases in blood that often happen when people get older.

The evidence shows that about 80 percent of the people with normal blood pressure, which is 120/80 mm Hg, are not sensitive. Of those who suffer from prehypertension, which is a precursor to hypertension, about 75 percent are not sensitive to salt.

Some of the health benefits of salt include:

- Helps prevent dehydration
- Helps with bone health
- Aids with digestion and nutrient absorption
- Maintains proper electrolyte balance
- Maintains proper pH balance in the body
- Helps with adrenal function
- Helps with regulation of blood pressure
- Helps with proper muscle function
- Aids with nutrient transport
- Helps with brain and nerve Function
- Saline solutions for breaking up phlegm in throat and wound cleaning
- Necessary for cell-to-cell communication
- Helps the heart pump blood throughout the body

What happens when you restrict your salt intake? You open yourself up to various health risks, such as increased heart risk, higher triglycerides, higher insulin levels, hypothyroidism, adrenal insufficiency, compromised functioning of the kidneys, obesity, insulin resistance, and type 2 diabetes.

Chronic salt depletion can lead to what is called internal starvation. Your body begins to panic when you start restricting your salt intake. One of the things that the body starts doing is increasing its insulin levels. This happens so that the kidney retains more sodium. Elevated insulin levels will lock energy into your fat cells. This means you will have trouble breaking down stored protein into amino acids or fat into fatty acids. The only macronutrient that can now utilize energy efficiently is carbohydrate.

What happens now is you begin to crave refined carbs and sugar like crazy. This is because your body thinks your only dependable energy source is carbohydrates. You eat more refined carbs, and you crave them more. The cycle keeps repeating itself where you overeat sugar and refined carbs and keep craving them.

Eventually, this will lead to insulin resistance, weight gain, and eventually type 2 diabetes.

The real culprit is not salt but sugar. Salt may be the solution instead of the cause of some chronic diseases affecting millions of people.

We would be fine if we eliminated or at least greatly reduced sugar from our diets. If we eliminated salt from our diets, we would die. Scientists have observed that sodium deficiency can lead to cannibalism in insects.

Salt helps with reproduction. It was known in Ancient Greece that animals that ate a lot of salt produced more milk and that salt made animals more eager to mate.

Farmers see similar things with today's livestock. Reducing sodium levels leads to smaller birth weights and litter size. Reducing the salt level also decreased the successful mating in female pigs. Sodium deficiency also brought about reproduction failure in mice. Low-salt diets reduce sex drive as well as the possibility of getting pregnant, as well as the weight of infants, sleep problems, and fatigue.

The founding editor of the Journal of Hypertension, Dr. John D. Swales, who was also a hypertension expert, published a paper in 2000 about salt. That paper showed that people with normal blood pressure get only a tiny reduction in systolic blood pressure (1 to 2 mmHg) and diastolic blood pressure (0.1 to 1 mmHg) when their sodium intake is severely restricted.

Dr. James DiNicolantonio writes in his book, *The Salt Fix: Why the Experts Got It All Wrong - And How Eating More Might Save Your*

Life, "Three countries with the lowest rate of death due to coronary heart disease in the world (Japan, France, and South Korea) all eat a very high-salt diet. The Mediterranean diet, the eating pattern now widely recommended as a heart-healthy diet, is quite high in salt (think sardines and anchovies, olives and capers, aged cheese, soups, shellfish, and goat's milk)... Norway eats more salt than the United States yet has a lower rate of death due to coronary heart disease. Even Switzerland and Canada have very low rates of death due to stroke despite a high-salt diet."

Dr. DiNicolantonio continues, "The bottom line is that even in countries known for eating a lot of salt, coronary heart disease also seems to be the lowest among those that consume the highest amounts of sodium. Among women in Korea, for example, the group consuming the highest amounts of sodium has a 13.5 percent lower prevalence of hypertension compared to the group consuming the lowest amounts of sodium. And at least fourteen countries consume a diet high in salt but have a low rate of death due to coronary heart disease. All of these countries consume the same amount of salt as people in the United States, if not more, and yet have a lower rate of death due to coronary heart disease."

So you can see that despite for many decades being told that salt raises blood pressure and the risk of heart attacks and strokes, it's clear that is simply not the case. We see that increasing salt intake reduces the risk of heart disease and premature death.

People with normal blood pressure have been known to excrete up to ten times the normal sodium intake, up to 86 grams of salt excreted per day.

Many people seem to ignore the fact that diabetics are known to likely have elevated blood pressure as well.

High cortisol levels also cause hypertension. Guess what leads to higher cortisol levels? It is not salt but sugar.

Many populations that eat a high-salt diet don't have hypertension. The same can't be said for those populations eating lots of sugar.

Lowering salt intake has been shown to speed up arteries' hardening and increase triglycerides and cholesterol in animals.

The so-called bad cholesterol (LDL) was found to increase in people with chronic high blood pressure who decreased their salt intake.

Many people don't know that the famous DASH-Sodium trail, which is the foundation of the best-known low-salt diet, actually discovered that restricting salt increases LDL and triglycerides.

People who had normal blood pressure and normal weight on low-salt diets have been shown to experience reduced good cholesterol (HDL), compromised kidney function, and lower levels of adiponectin, which is a substance that fat cells release that improves insulin sensitivity.

Salt restriction increases the heart rate. This matters because the heart will receive blood supply while it is relaxing. The other organs get blood while the heart is contracting. When the heart beats and pumps faster, it has less time to relax and receive blood and oxygen. With the blood flow reduced to the heart now as a result of the low-salt diet, that can increase the risk of heart attacks.

One hundred thousand people in seventeen countries were examined in the Prospective Urban Rural Epidemiology Study. They discovered that the lowest risk of cardiovascular events and death was in people who consumed between 3,000 and 6,000 milligrams of sodium each day. The great risk of cardiovascular events and death was in those who consumed less than 3,000 milligrams of sodium per day.

Not only have low-salt diets been found to increase insulin levels and insulin resistance, but they have also been linked to nonalcoholic fatty liver disease, also called fatty liver disease.

Caffeine increases the excretion of salt. People who exercise a lot and athletes may lose up to two grams of salt in an hour.

Various studies show that low-salt diets may cause anxiety and hypochondriasis. The University of Haifa in Israel, in a 2011 study, suggests that higher consumption of salt can help reduce stress.

Low-salt diets can reduce the amount of total water in the body and cause dehydration.

Low-salt diets can lead to sodium depletion, which can weaken muscle strength and energy metabolism because of the increase in the acidity of the cells.

Increasing your salt intake can help with arthritis.

Low-salt diets also lead to decreased energy and increased fatigue.

Try to make sure you get enough salt in your diet and enjoy!

Chapter 16
Why Enzymes are Important for your Health

Enzymes are catalysts that help speed up the rate of chemical reactions in our bodies. They are usually proteins but can also be RNAs (which are known as ribozymes).

Enzymes are important for digestion, respiration, muscle and nerve function, liver function, essential for digestion, and much more.

The length of our lives is proportional to the amount of enzymes we have. More enzymes mean longer life. Enzymes carry the life force in the body.

Enzymes pull things together. It's a catalyst. Catalysts speed up the rate of reaction.

Metabolic Enzymes are enzymes that make things happen. They improve health.

Digestive Enzymes are enzymes that make digestion happen. They pull foods apart. They also help increase nutrient absorption. They spare the metabolic enzymes.

Digestive enzymes require the proper PH level in the stomach. There must be acid in the stomach. Take digestive enzymes with acid.

When you run out of one enzyme, the other enzyme will compensate for it. If you lose digestive enzymes, the metabolic enzymes will replace them, and you will eventually run out of metabolic enzymes. This will make you age quicker and get worse. Food enzymes will help spare metabolic enzymes.

Vitamins are coenzymes. They support enzymatic activity.

Enzymes are only in living food. They can't be added to enriched foods.

The more you cook the food, the more enzymes are destroyed. Raw fruits and vegetables carry the life force. Lack of enzymes is a major cause of illness.

Food Enzymes assist digestive enzymes, so you spare the metabolic enzymes.

Betaine Hydrochloride helps with methylation.

The ending "ase" refers to enzymes. Protease breaks down proteins. Lipase breaks down fats and lipids. Amylase breaks down carbohydrates.

Lack of enzymes speeds up the aging process.

Enzyme deficiencies with digestive enzymes will make it harder to break down foods, particularly proteins. Proteins will not break down into amino acids but will remain as peptides if you don't get enough enzymes.

The immune system is always on the lookout for peptides to see if the enemy has invaded the body. Peptides trigger immune reactions if not broken down. This is the cause of many autoimmune and inflammation issues. Enemy foreign peptides are perceived to have gotten into the blood, activating the immune system. Complete breakdown of proteins is very important to prevent immune activation.

Proteases break down proteins in the blood. Proteins in the blood take the form of clotting and fibrin formation. Proteases are anti-clotting and thin the blood.

Digestive enzymes also have anti-pain properties. Digestive enzymes taken on an empty stomach can speed healing, especially after surgery.

The pancreas is an enzyme factory. It's where most of the enzymes are made. When the pancreas gets cancer, you don't make enzymes.

One of the reasons pancreatic cancer is so deadly is that enzymes come from the pancreas.

Enzymes can also explode throughout the body when you have pancreatic damage.

Pancreatic enzymes have a digestive effect in the enzymes, but instead of depending on acid, they depend on alkaline/non-acid.

Bile is alkaline and changes the pH of the chyme, which allows the pancreatic enzymes to enter the intestine. Chyme is the pulpy acid that passes from the stomach to the small intestine, consisting of gastric juices and partly digested food.

Pancreatic enzymes have been used for cystic fibrosis and cancer. Enzymes help with longevity, and they go to the intestine. Enzymes also help with pain, blood flow, speed up healing, and intestinal flow.

The more processed food you eat, the harder your body has to work to digest it.

Until recently, when we ate food, we also ate enzymes. That is no longer the case much of the time. When we cook our food, we lose our enzymes. Ultra-processed foods don't have enzymes.

Chapter 17
Eggs are Actually Healthy and Good for You

Eggs are one of the healthiest foods you can eat. Eggs have been eaten for breakfast for a long time. Unfortunately, eggs have gotten a bad reputation over the last several decades because they contain high levels of cholesterol. Eggs have some of the highest nutrient content out there. Eggs will have Vitamin D, various B Vitamins, Choline, Inositol, Selenium, Iodine, Vitamin E (sometimes), Zinc, Vitamin A, Iodine, Proteins, and EFAs. Eggs also have some trace minerals in them as well. Some people only eat the egg white because egg yolks have cholesterol and egg whites don't and also have protein. The problem is that most other nutrients are in the egg yolk, not the egg white. And almost 40% of the proteins are also in the egg yolk. People who eat eggs daily don't have their cholesterol levels go up.

Eggs also contain the antioxidants zeaxanthin and lutein. These two important antioxidants vanquish free radicals that may accumulate in your eyes and thus protect your vision. They also thwart cataracts.

Eggs also aid in myelin sheath repair. Myelin is a sheath that insulates and protects your nerves. It also transmits electrical impulses, which help your body function.

Eating eggs has a lot of benefits.

Whole eggs are nutritionally rich, supplying almost every nutrient you need. They are useful sources of nutrients like vitamins D and B12 as well as the mineral iodine. Eggs are regarded as a 'complete' source of protein as they contain the essential amino acids that we must obtain from our diet.

Furthermore, if you choose brands enriched with omega-3 fattys acids, due to the diet the chickens are fed, you'll benefit from higher omega-3 fatty acids as well as fat-soluble vitamins such as vitamins A and E.

Eggs are really among the most nutritious foods on the planet.

A single large boiled egg contains:

- Vitamin A: 8% of the DV (daily value)
- Folate (Vitamin B9): 6% of the DV
- Pantothenic acid (vitamin B5): 14% of the DV
- Vitamin B12: 23% of the DV
- Riboflavin (Vitamin B2): 20% of the DV
- Phosphorus: 7% of the DV
- Selenium: 28% of the DV

- Eggs also contain decent amounts of vitamin D, E, B6, Calcium, and zinc.

This comes with 78 calories, 6 grams of protein, and 5 grams of fat. Eggs also contain various trace nutrients that are important for health.

In fact, eggs are pretty much the perfect food. They contain a little bit of almost every nutrient you need.

Eggs are rich in several nutrients that promote heart health, such as betaine and choline. A study of nearly half a million people in China suggests that eating one egg a day may reduce the risk of heart disease and stroke.

One egg delivers around 207 milligrams of cholesterol, about 69% of the daily limit recommended by the Dietary Guidelines for Americans. For those of you who worry about too much cholesterol, the truth is that eating dietary cholesterol does not directly correlate to making your blood cholesterol levels go up, and dietary cholesterol has just a tiny impact on our blood cholesterol levels.

One of the reasons eggs have pretty much no effect on heart disease risk is that eggs help raise high-density lipoprotein (HDL) levels – aka "good" cholesterol.

Eggs are also a great source of heart-healthy nutrients like folate and other B vitamins. According to other research, eating two eggs per day improves heart health.

The yolk of the egg is a source of important nutrients like vitamin D, vitamin B12, and choline, which are vital for helping our bodies process food into energy we can use. Also, the combination of protein and healthy fat will help you feel full for longer.

Eggs are an excellent source of B vitamins such as vitamins B2, B5, and B12. These B vitamins help maintain healthy skin and hair in addition to other functions. Eggs are also a good source of amino acids like methionine, which can help enhance the tone and flexibility of the skin as well as the sturdiness of nails and hair.

Eggs are a good source of choline, an important nutrient necessary for everyone to produce cell membranes and vital neurotransmitters in the body and for brain function and memory. Choline is crucial during breastfeeding and pregnancy because normal brain development requires a sufficient supply of choline. Choline is vital for heart health and supports the brain, nerves, liver, muscle control, general nervous function, memory, and mood. You will probably be able to think more clearly. You might be able to think more clearly because of the choline in eggs.

A deficiency can lead to various symptoms, such as brain fog. You get about 6% of your daily choline needs from eating one egg, and so a healthy brain can be supported by eating eggs.

Choline in eggs helps repair myelin and aids in myelin regrowth.

Eggs may support eye health. That is because the egg yolk has sizable amounts of carotenoids, in particular zeaxanthin and lutein. These two are crucial for defending against cataracts and macular degeneration. Eggs also have vitamin A, which is beneficial for good eyesight and helps prevent macular degeneration.

Eggs are very filling and score high on the satiety index, which is a measure of how filling a food is. It has been demonstrated in studies that an egg breakfast is more filling and sustaining than a carb breakfast with the equivalent calorie count. And that egg breakfast may help decrease your calorie intake later in the day.

Eggs are a great and nutritious source of vitamins, minerals, proteins, and essential fatty acids, especially in the yolk. About 60 percent of the protein is found in the egg white, and this helps you feel full and can assist you in managing your weight.

Eggs are one of the best food options to help manage your weight since they are a great source of protein and have relatively low calories. The high satiety levels of eggs will make you feel less hungry, more satisfied, and a lower desire to reach that midday snack.

Eating eggs can make you feel full longer for several reasons. It boosts metabolic activity. It also raises your hormone leptin level, which helps you feel satisfied and not hungry after you eat. Eating eggs will also keep your energy levels high and will slow down the rate at which food will leave your stomach.

Eggs are also a good source of leucine. Leucine is an amino acid that is important for muscle protein synthesis. It also supports muscle health and exercise recovery.

In eggs, the combination of choline, tryptophan, choline, vitamin B2, and B12 are all associated with helping lessen the symptoms of depression and risk of anxiety and naturally helping with sleep.

Vitamin D helps us maintain healthy and strong bones by improving calcium absorption in the gut. Vitamin D also aids in keeping our calcium and phosphorus levels in a range that promotes healthy bone remodeling and bone growth. About 6% of our Vitamin D needs are provided by eating one egg, so adding a couple of eggs to your plate each day can help your bones reap benefits.

So what happened?

Eggs get a bad rap because of their high cholesterol content. There is a lot of cholesterol in the yolk. People were told to limit the number of eggs they eat, and some people would not eat the yolk but only eat the white egg. By not eating the egg yolk, they are missing out on a lot of nutrition, as the yolk is where most of the nutrition is. The egg white has a lot of protein, which is fine, but many people don't know that almost 40% of the protein in the egg is actually in the yolk.

Eggs have been eaten for many centuries and are one of the healthiest things to eat for breakfast. Nowadays, people will eat croissants, bagels, or cereal for breakfast, all of which have lots of carbs, which is detrimental to your health.

If you want to improve your health, consider adding eggs to your diet.

Chapter 18
Why Having Enough Stomach Acid is Vital for Good Health

Many people don't realize the importance of having enough stomach acid. They think having too much of it is bad for their health. Most people think that acid reflux is caused by too much acid. It's actually the opposite. It's caused by too little acid. Usually, around the age of 35, most people start producing less stomach acid. It is usually in your late 30s that you start experiencing more heartburn and acid reflux. Now, since you are producing less stomach acid as you start getting older, how can acid reflux be caused by too much stomach acid? If too much acid was the problem, then teenagers would have lots of acid reflux problems, while grandma and grandpa would have little acid reflux problems. Of course, we know that teenagers rarely get acid reflux, while it is far more common in older people.

You will get some temporary relief if you take medicines, antacids, and bases to deal with acid reflux. But you are reducing the amount of stomach acid, and with less stomach acid, you will be able to absorb fewer nutrients. You also open yourself up to more diseases as stomach acid kills bacteria and pathogens that can harm you. One reason you should avoid drinking carbonated drinks is that they will also reduce stomach acid. Again, this will lead to your inability to absorb nutrients as well.

The other thing is that once you stop taking the antacid medicines, the condition will return, and you will feel acid reflux.

Taking an antacid for occasional use can reduce heartburn and not do any real harm. Long-term use can lead to all kinds of damages. In addition to being unable to absorb nutrients, it can also lead to milk-alkali syndrome, the symptoms of which are an elevated blood pH (aka alkalosis), excess calcium in your blood, and kidney failure. Milk-Alkali Syndrome results from excessive consumption of milk (which has calcium) and antacids over a prolonged period or occurs by taking excessive calcium-based acid neutralizers for a long time.

Heartburn itself rarely signals too much acid but usually too little. When they measure the stomach acid output of heartburn sufferers, the overwhelming majority of them have too little stomach acid production.

These acid-reducing medicines and antacids also disrupt the gastrointestinal environment. They lead to profound changes in the internal environment of the intestines and stomach. They also don't cure heartburn. They only temporarily relieve the symptoms.

What should you do then? You need to get more acid in your stomach. There are a couple of ways to do this. You can start taking betaine hydrochloride tablets with pepsin.

You can also start taking apple cider vinegar tablets. Apple cider vinegar has acetic acid, which helps increase the acid in your stomach. I recommend taking the tablets over the liquid.

You don't want less stomach acid in your body. You want more stomach acid in the body. If you have less stomach acid, you won't be able to absorb nutrients either. This malabsorption of nutrients can lead to a whole bunch of conditions such as arthritis, depression, osteoporosis, and other chronic degenerative diseases that lessen your quality of life as well as possibly shorten your life.

Having enough acid in the stomach is crucial for properly absorbing minerals from our food, killing unwanted organisms (such as viruses, yeast, parasites, bacteria, and fungi) that can get into our water and food, and proper digestion of protein.

Acid is in your stomach because it is supposed to be there. It is important for the digestive process; without stomach acid, our digestive and overall health will suffer.

Many studies going back to the early 1900s have linked gallbladder disease with low secretion of stomach acid.

Most autoimmune conditions often have low levels of stomach acid present.

They have known since the 1920s that low stomach acid occurs disproportionately in people suffering from numerous diseases.

Children with asthma often have low stomach acid and Vitamin B12. Once they get more stomach acid and B12, their conditions improve.

Most bacteria cannot survive long in a very acidic environment such as the stomach. When the stomach becomes less and less acidic, that all changes. Some bacteria that survive in a less acidic stomach environment may not do too much damage. They may interfere with the digestion of nutrients and cause symptoms like constipation, diarrhea, and even some stomach pain. However, some microorganisms, such as some virulent strains of E. Coli, Salmonella, Cholera, Dysentery, Typhoid, and Tuberculosis, can lead to very serious illness and even to death sometimes. All this happens due to very low stomach acid in the stomach.

The market for antacids and acid-reducing drugs is huge. The global antacid market hit $14 billion in 2023 and is expected to go up to $22 billion. That is a lot of money.

Chapter 19
Why You Should be Exercising

Exercise is one of the best things you can do for your health. You definitely want to make sure you get enough exercise and are not living a sedentary lifestyle.

<u>There are lots of benefits to exercising. They include:</u>

- Helps improve your brain health. One of the benefits of exercise is improved cognition or thinking for kids between the ages of 6 to 13. Exercise also helps your brain remain sharp as you age. It can help you sleep better. Exercise can also lower your risk of anxiety and depression. I can tell you from personal experience that taking a nice, long walk relaxes, destresses and helps me feel better.
- Assist you in controlling your weight. In addition to diet, exercise is very important in preventing obesity and managing your weight.
- Exercise improves your circulation and strengthens your heart. Oxygen levels go up because of the increased blood flow. This helps decrease your risk of coronary artery disease and heart attack. Exercising regularly can decrease your blood pressure and triglyceride levels.
- Exercise can reduce your blood sugar level and it can also help your insulin work better. This can decrease your risk for type 2 diabetes and metabolic syndrome.
- Exercise can reduce your cravings as well as withdrawal symptoms, which can help make it easier to quit smoking. It helps you feel better, bolster your mood, and improve your mental health. Chemicals are released by your body that can help you feel more relaxed and help better your mood while you're exercising. This can lower your risk of depression as well as help you handle stress better.
- Exercise causes your body to release chemicals and proteins that enhance the function and structure of your brain. This will aid in keeping your learning, thinking, and judgment skills sharp as you get older.
- Exercising regularly can help children and teens develop big, strong bones. It can also delay the bone density loss that

occurs with aging. Performing muscle-strengthening activities may help you maintain or increase muscle size and strength.

- Lessens your risk of some cancers, such as lung, uterine, breast, and colon cancer.
- Older adults usually have higher risks of falling. Various research shows that performing muscle-strengthening and balance activities and doing mild-intensity aerobic activity can help decrease the risk of falling for older people.
- Exercise can enhance your sexual health. The risk of erectily dysfunction (ED) in men may be reduced by exercising regularly. Exercise may increase sexual arousal in women.
- Improve your chances of longevity. Various studies show that physical activity can improve your chances of living longer and decrease your risk of dying early from heart disease and some cancers.

Exercise increases your energy
Exercise and physical activity will increase your endurance and improve your muscle strength. Exercising delivers nutrients and oxygen to the tissues and helps the cardiovascular system work more smoothly and effectively. You will have greater energy to handle daily chores when your lungs and heart health get better.
Exercise supports and promotes better sleep
If you are having trouble sleeping, then regular physical activity and exercise will help you fall asleep more quickly and stay asleep longer. Try not to exercise near your bedtime as you may have trouble sleeping as you will have too much energy to fall asleep.

Other benefits of exercise include:

1. Decreases Cancer Risk
2. Reduces Stress
3. Cleans Arteries
4. Helps Manage Chronic Pain
5. Oxygenates the Body
6. Increases your lifespan
7. Improves Coordination
8. Improves Complexion
9. Lessen Blood Pressure
10. Wards off viruses

Exercising and being physically active are wonderful ways to improve your mood, feel better, have fun, and improve your health. Exercising regularly is beneficial to the gut and can help protect it. Exercising and working out may encourage the growth of healthy microbiomes in your gut. Working out can increase levels of the bacterial metabolite butyrate, which helps promote gut barrier integrity.

Exercise can reduce the inflammation in your body.

Exercising also helps drop the uric acid levels in the body. Uric acid has been linked to a whole bunch of diseases, such as heart disease, kidney disease, fatty liver disease, diabetes, metabolic syndrome, and high blood pressure. High uric acid can also damage the ligaments, tendons, joints, and bones.

Exercising also fosters balanced hormones.

While exercise has a lot of great benefits, one thing to keep in mind is that when you are exercising, you are also sweating out vitamins and minerals. So, after you are done exercising, you need to replenish the vitamins and minerals to avoid becoming deficient in them. If you exercise and don't replace the vitamins and minerals you sweat out, it will cause a lot of health problems. Exercise without supplementation is suicide.

One of the reasons you sometimes hear about a star high school athlete dropping dead during practice is because while he was practicing and exercising on the field, he was sweating out all those vitamins and minerals and was not replacing them and became deficient in them, and it eventually caught up to him, and led to his death. It is one of the reasons young star athletes pass away.

Exercise has lots of great benefits and can undo some of the damage caused by eating bad foods. Unfortunately, you can't outrun a bad diet, and exercise won't address all of the health issues caused by a bad diet. Exercising by itself will not improve oxidative stress, nor will it improve glycation or membrane fluidity and integrity. Just something to remember about exercising. Still, there are a lot of great benefits to exercising, as has already been mentioned.

Exercise helps make more and fresh mitochondria. It can also help improve your skin health.

Make sure to find time to exercise. Your body and health will thank you for it.

Chapter 20
The Awesome Benefits of CoQ10

CoQ10 is a very important nutrient for your health.
When you have low levels of CoQ10 levels, a number of diseases have been linked to CoQ10 deficiency, such as Heart Failure, Diabetes, Alzheimer's disease, Migraines, and Cancer.
CoQ10 helps with heart disease and helps people who suffer from congestive heart failure. It also helps with angina. It also helps with arrhythmia as it has a stabilizing effect on the heart. CoQ10 also helps prevent atherosclerosis (hardening of the arteries). CoQ10 helps with high blood pressure. Various research indicates CoQ10 may improve treatment outcomes for heart failure patients.
CoQ10 can help bring back optimal levels of energy production, improve heart function, and lessen oxidative damage. All of these can help treat heart failure.
A review of 14 studies discovered that heart failure patients who were supplemented with CoQ10 supplements had a reduced risk of dying as well as a bigger improvement in exercise capacity compared to those patients who took a placebo.
COQ10 may improve heart health, and CoQ10 can be helpful for cardiac cells as they have high energy requirements, and low levels of CoQ10 adversely affect them. By boosting the availability of nitric oxide, CoQ10 can promote the widening of the blood vessels and lower blood pressure.
A review of people who suffered from heart failure showed that supplementing with CoQ10 led to improvements in heart function, fewer hospitalizations, and a decreased risk of death.
CoQ10 may help fight certain types of cancer and may also play a role in cancer prevention. Some test-tube studies show that CoQ10 may block the growth of cancer cells. It has been noted that people who suffer from cancer often have lower levels of CoQ10. Various older studies suggest having lower levels of CoQ10 correlated with increases in some forms of cancer, such as prostate and breast cancer. Some newer studies suggest the same increased risk in regard to lung cancer for those with low CoQ10 levels.
CoQ10 can help sufferers of Chronic Fatigue Syndrome
Statins are drugs that are given to help lower cholesterol. One side effect is they can lower the COQ10 levels. This can cause muscle pain and weakness as a side effect. Statins can also cause cramps. CoQ10 can help reduce these side effects of muscle pain,

weakness, and cramps. If you are taking statins, your COQ10 levels very often go down while taking the statins. Using a good COQ10 supplement to offset the COQ10 you may lose using the statins is a good idea.

CoQ10 reduces oxidative stress, which can also support heart health. Oxidative stress has been suggested as a contributing factor to both Parkinson's and Alzheimer's disease. CoQ10 supplementation has been suggested to reduce the progression of these diseases by decreasing oxidative stress.

CoQ10 can help those suffering from diabetes. CoQ10 may help improve diabetes. Since CoQ10 is an antioxidant that decreases oxidative stress, supplementing with it may help decrease insulin resistance in people suffering from diabetes.

Consistently high levels of blood sugar lead to insulin resistance as well as produce oxidative stress. Insulin is a hormone that lowers your blood sugar. When you become insulin resistant, the body does not use insulin efficiently, which raises blood sugar levels.

One of the main factors in type 2 diabetes is insulin resistance. CoQ10 seems to improve insulin sensitivity and regulate blood sugar levels, according to a 2018 meta-analysis.

According to a study done with people who suffer from diabetic neuropathy, which is a type of nerve damage that happens in diabetes sufferers discovered that by taking 100 mg of CoQ10 daily for three months, they may have improvements in insulin resistance and HbA1c levels, as well as decreased markers of oxidative stress.

Supplementing with CoQ10 supplementation may improve blood sugar control in people with type 2 diabetes, improve HDL cholesterol, and lower triglycerides.

CoQ10 may help reduce migraines. People who have experienced painful migraine headaches often have low levels of CoQ10.

A review of people with migraines discovered that supplementing at least six with CoQ10 decreased the length and frequency of migraines, although it did not lessen the migraine pain. CoQ10 can reduce headaches. Low energy in the brain cells can occur from abnormal mitochondrial function, and this can contribute to migraines.

CoQ10 may be beneficial for the treatment of migraines since it lives mainly in the mitochondria of cells. Several studies show that CoQ10 can lessen the frequency and duration of migraines in both adults and children.

CoQ10 may help slow skin aging. CoQ10 reduces the number of free radicals that may lead to wrinkles in the skin. There is also some evidence suggesting that CoQ10 applied to the skin in creams may help fight the visible signs of aging.

CoQ10 may also improve athletic performance, as several studies suggest CoQ10 can help improve exercise recovery and delay fatigue.

CoQ10 can be found naturally in your body, in some foods, and supplements.

Food Sources of CoQ10 include meat, fish, nuts, and some oils. The body makes some CoQ10, but in amounts that are much less than what has been shown in studies to be beneficial.

Your body produces CoQ10, but your CoQ10 levels decline as you get older. This leads to lessening your body's ability to control oxidative stress and inflammation effectively.

CoQ10 may help with fertility.

As women get older, their fertility decreases as a result of the decline in the number and quality of available eggs. CoQ10 production slows as you get older, which makes the body less effective at shielding the eggs from oxidative damage. CoQ10 supplementation helps and might even reverse the age-related decline in egg quantity and quality.

Male sperm is also susceptible to oxidative damage. This can cause decreased sperm count, infertility, and substandard sperm quality.

Various studies have indicated that CoQ10 supplementation can improve sperm quality, concentration, and activity by increasing antioxidant protection.

Applying CoQ10 cream to the skin can promote antioxidant protection, may help decrease oxidative damage caused by UV rays, and lessen the depth of wrinkles, according to various animal and human studies.

Abnormal mitochondrial function may decrease muscle energy. This will make it more difficult for the muscles to efficiently contract as well as to sustain exercise.

CoQ10 reduces oxidative stress in your cells and improves mitochondrial function, which can aid with exercise performance. Taking CoQ10 supplements may help lessen fatigue.

As you get older, your mitochondrial function usually decreases. This decrease of mitochondria can cause the death of brain cells, which can lead to diseases such as Parkinson's and Alzheimer's.

The brain is susceptible to oxidative stress because of its high demand for oxygen and its high fatty acid composition.

Oxidative stress supports the production of dangerous substances that could alter and affect physical, memory, and cognition functions.

CoQ10 may be able to reduce these dangerous substances and possibly slow down the advancement of Parkinson's and Alzheimer's disease, according to several animal studies.

Lung diseases such as asthma and COPD (chronic obstructive pulmonary disease) can occur as a result of increased oxidative damage in the lungs, low levels of CoQ10, and poor antioxidant protection.

Some older studies have discovered that people with lung diseases often have lower levels of CoQ10.

Make sure to get enough CoQ10 in your diet.

Chapter 21
Vitamin A

Vitamin A is one of the four fat-soluble vitamins, with vitamins D, E and K. Fat soluble means it can dissolve in fats and oils. These fat-soluble vitamins are absorbed along with fats in your diet and are stored in the liver and the body's fatty (adipose) tissue for future use, unlike water-soluble vitamins. Fat-soluble vitamins are better absorbed if eaten with fat.

Beta Carotene is actually a precursor to Vitamin A. Vitamin A helps improve your immune system. It is a powerful antioxidant and helps fight against free radicals.

Vitamin A is also extremely important for your skin. Vitamin A helps with acne. In fact, Accutane, which is often used to treat acne, is a synthetic version of Vitamin A.

Vitamin A eye drops may help with dry eyes. Vitamin A deficiency can lead to dry eyes.

Vitamin A can help people with AIDS. One thing many people who are HIV positive have in common is that they are vitamin A deficient. Vitamin A has been shown to improve immune function and increase the concentration of CD4 T-cells in the body.

Vitamin A may help with night blindness.

Vitamin A is helpful for respiratory tract infections like bronchitis. It aids in improving immune function against viral infections.

Vitamin A may help lower your risk of some forms of cancer.

Vitamin A helps the brain and the nervous system. Children need adequate amounts of Vitamin A so they can learn properly.

Food Sources of Vitamin A include:

- Beef liver
- Carrots
- Sweet Potatoes
- Broccoli
- Milk and dairy
- Squash
- Parsley
- Kale
- Spinach
- Salmon
- Trout

- Chicken Liver
- Cod Liver Oil
- Cantaloupe
- Papaya
- Mango

Vitamin A deficiencies can lead to:

- Eye inflammation
- Night Blindness
- Decreased resistance to infection
- Improper tooth and bone formation
- Weight loss
- Skin Irritation
- Issues with Fertility
- Stunted Growth
- Acne
- Dermatitis
- Immune System Issues
- Increased Risk of Cancer
- Depression

Chapter 22
Vitamin B (B Complex Vitamins)

The various B vitamins are best taken together, which is where we get the term "B-Complex." They are extremely important for our health.

Vitamin B is a water-soluble vitamin. Water soluble means that it can be dissolved in water. The difference between water-soluble and fat-soluble is that water-soluble vitamins are carried to the body's tissues, but they are not stored in the body, unlike fat-soluble vitamins. Water-soluble vitamins must be taken every day and replenished.

Since water-soluble vitamins are dissolved in water, your body will get rid of anything that is not needed in your urine. If these water-soluble vitamins are not adequately replaced, nutritional deficiencies and health problems can occur.

Thiamine (B1)

Vitamin B1 helps convert food into energy. Vitamin B1 is necessary to metabolize fats, proteins, and carbohydrates. It breaks down carbohydrates for energy.

Thiamine is a powerful antioxidant and helps prevent wrinkles and age spots.

Thiamine B1 is important for your immune system and can help protect your brain, heart, and nervous system.

Thiamine is important for promoting digestion as it is required for the secretion of hydrochloric acid, which is necessary for the total digestion of food particles.

B1 can help boost energy. It can also improve mood and prevent depression.

Vitamin B1 helps to make adenosine triphosphate (ATP). This is very important as all your body's cells use and store ATP for energy.

B1 can also help prevent cataracts. It can also help with blood sugar control, as Type 1 and Type 2 diabetics often have low levels of thiamine.

B1 can also help prevent complications in the stomach and intestines.

B1 supports muscle contractions and movements of signals in the brain.

B1 can help improve appetite and prevent Alzheimer's disease.

Alcoholics are often prone to a vitamin B1 deficiency. Drinking alcohol will, over time, decrease B1 absorption through the intestines. You need B1 to metabolize alcohol. Alcohol causes B1 deficiency and can lead to eye movement issues and permanent memory impairment. It can also lead to Wenicke's encephalopathy, where damage to the brain and psychosis can happen.
Antibiotics can also deplete your B1 levels.
Vitamin B1 may also help prevent cataracts.
Sundowner's Syndrome affects the elderly and is similar to Alzheimer's disease. It's caused by a vitamin B1 deficiency. If you get them Vitamin B1, it will mostly be back to normal in a couple of weeks.

Deficiencies in Thiamin (B1) can lead to:

- Nausea
- Anorexia
- Depression
- Muscular Weakness
- Paralysis
- Short-term Memory Loss
- Peripheral Neuropathies
- Beriberi
- Mental Confusion
- Anxiety
- Headaches
- Abdominal Discomfort
- Sundowner's Syndrome

Food sources of Thiamine (B1) include:
- Eggs
- Salmon
- Trout
- Lentils
- Pork
- Beef
- Yogurt
- Black Beans
- Sunflower Seeds
- Organ Meats
- Whole Grain Foods
- Potatoes

Riboflavin (B2)

Vitamin B2 (riboflavin) has been shown to lessen the duration and frequency of migraine headaches. Riboflavin is also important for cell energy production. Vitamin B2 may also help prevent cataracts.

Riboflavin also works as an antioxidant and fights free radicals. Riboflavin also helps make adenosine triphosphate (ATP). ATP is very important for storing energy in muscles.

Vitamin B2 also helps with brain and heart health. Riboflavin also supports your growth and development.

Deficiencies in Vitamin B2 can lead to:

- Anemia
- Neuropathy
- Lacrimation (or Tearing)
- Slowed Growth
- Digestive Problems
- Sensitivity to Light
- Cracks at the corners of the mouth and nostrils (Cheilosis)
- Burning and soreness of the mouth, tongue and lips

Food sources of Vitamin B2 include:

- Eggs
- Green Leafy Vegetables
- Organ Meats
- Cheese
- Yogurt
- Dairy
- Whole Grains
- Salmon
- Almonds

Niacin (B3)

Vitamin B3 (Niacin) is such an important vitamin that if a severe deficiency occurs, the body will make niacin. Niacin is also being used to treat Social Anxiety Disorder.

Niacin is important for cardiovascular health. Niacin is a vasodilator. It opens up the blood vessels, making niacin a great anti-hypertensive that lowers blood pressure.

Niacin helps improve circulation and helps convert nutrients into energy.

For those concerned about their cholesterol levels, niacin is great at lowering cholesterol.

Niacin also helps slow the progression of dementia.

In a 2022 study at the Indiana University School of Medicine that was published in Science Translational Magazine, researchers discovered that niacin limits the progression of Alzheimer's disease when used in models in the lab.

Another study in the Journal of Neurology, Neurosurgery, and Psychiatry looked at niacin intake and Alzheimer's disease occurrence in over 6,000 people. The results from the researchers showed that the people with the highest totals of niacin were far less likely to develop Alzheimer's disease than those who took the lower totals. According to the same study, a big food intake of niacin corresponded with a slower rate of cognitive decline.

The niacin benefits for dementia arise from the fact that niacin is important for antioxidant functions in the brain, formation and growth of nerve cells, cell signaling, and DNA synthesis and repair.

Niacin is also one of the most effective ways to lower bad cholesterol and raise good cholesterol. There is no need to use statins or other drugs. Studies have shown that Niacin lowers LDL cholesterol by 10 to 25 percent and triglycerides by 20 to 50 percent.

When LDL cholesterol is lowered by niacin, there is a favorable reduction of the really vicious and nasty small and dense LDL particles that stick to the artery walls and oxidize and cause damage.

Niacin also decreases the level of lipoprotein(a) or Lp(a). Lipoprotein(a) is a really bad and nasty kind of LDL. Lipoprotein(a) is a risk factor for heart attacks and heart disease. However, little attention is paid to Lipoprotein(a) since no drug treatments lower it. However, niacin reduces Lipoprotein(a) levels by 10 to 30 percent.

Niacin also raises HDL cholesterol (aka the good cholesterol), and it raises it by 10 to 30 percent.

Signs of Niacin Deficiency include:

- Diarrhea
- Dermatitis
- Dementia
- Death
- Anorexia
- Skin pigmentation
- Muscular Weakness

Food sources of Niacin include:

- Anorexia
- Skin pigmentation
- Red meat: beef, beef liver, pork
- Turkey
- Chicken Breast
- Brown rice
- Nuts and seeds
- Legumes
- Bananas
- Salmon
- Tuna
- Avocado
- Mushrooms
- Green Peas
- Potatoes

Pantothenic Acid (B5)

Vitamin B5 is sometimes called the adrenal vitamin since the adrenal glands require Vitamin B5 to make stress hormones. When a person is under a lot of stress, B5 helps the adrenal glands make enough stress hormones like cortisol. Producing enough stress hormones enables the body to successfully handle stress. A lot of nutritional adrenal support supplements contain Vitamin B5 (pantothenic acid) combined with other supplements that support the adrenal glands, like ginseng and Vitamin C.

Vitamin B5 helps with allergies. It also helps with fatigue.

Deficiencies in Vitamin B5 can lead to:

- Dermatitis
- Muscle Cramps

- Anemia
- Anorexia
- Depression
- Insomnia
- Tachycardia
- Light-Headedness
- Gastrointestinal Issues
- Immune System Issues

Pyridoxine (B6)

Vitamin B6 is involved in the metabolism of amino acids. Vitamin B6 helps alleviate the symptoms of PMS.

Vitamin B6 also aids in reducing the risk of heart disease.

Vitamin B6 helps lower a toxic component of protein metabolism called homocysteine. This is an important factor in cardiovascular disease, as 10 percent of the country's cardiovascular risk can be attributed to homocysteine.

Vitamin B6 can help with diabetes, epilepsy, asthma, water retention, and morning sickness.

Vitamin B6 can help reduce the symptoms of carpal tunnel syndrome.

Deficiencies in Vitamin B6 can lead to:

- Nausea and Vomiting
- PMS (Premenstrual Syndrome)
- Carpal Tunnel Syndrome
- Ataxia (Instability and lack of coordination)
- Tourette's Syndrome
- Irritability
- Convulsions and Seizures
- Depression
- Mental Confusion

Biotin (Vitamin B7 or Vitamin H)

Biotin is known best for its benefits for hair and nails. It helps make nails thicker and has been used for dealing with hair loss and thinning hair.

Biotin helps with the skin as well as regulates metabolism. It also helps with nerve health and is important for a healthy pregnancy in women.

Some studies have shown that biotin can help improve blood sugar in both Type 1 and Type 2 diabetes. It has also been known to help diabetics dealing with peripheral neuropathy.

Deficiencies in Biotin can lead to:

- Eczema
- Hair Loss
- Fatigue
- Muscle Pain
- Weight Loss
- Insomnia
- Anorexia
- Depression
- Fatty liver
- Brittle Hair
- Loss of Appetite
- Nausea

Food sources of Biotin include:

- Brewer's Yeast
- Milk
- Cheese
- Eggs
- Soybeans
- Cauliflower
- Whole Wheat Product
- Mushrooms
- Fish
- Nuts
- Liver and other organ meats

Folate or 'folic acid' acid when included in supplements (B9)
Vitamin B9 (folic acid) is very important for the brain. It helps those who suffer from poor memory and depression.
It also helps prevent defects in newborns, especially neural tube defects, which are incomplete brain and spinal cord development.
Folic acid is necessary for cell division.
Folic acid helps reduce the risk of colorectal cancer. It also lessens the risk of breast cancer in women.

Supplementation of Vitamin B9 can help with the symptoms of vitiligo. Gingivitis in pregnant women can be reduced by topically applying folic acid.

A Dutch three-year study found that supplementing with 800 mcg of folic acid daily slowed the rate of age-related hearing loss.

Deficiencies in Folic Acid (Vitamin B9) can lead to:

- Anemia
- Memory Issues
- Depression
- Gingivitis
- Other Health Issue

Methylcobalamin (B12)

Vitamin B12 is required for cell division.

Methylcobalamin (B12) versus cyanocobalamin (synthetic B12) - I recommend staying away from the synthetic form of B12 called cyanocobalamin and any supplements that have it. Use the natural form called Methylcobalamin.

B12 works with folic acid for many biochemical processes like the production of the myelin sheath and cell division.

B12 is often called the energy vitamin, and lots of people feel more energized after getting a B12 shot.

B12 also helps with depression, asthma, shingles, chronic fatigue, and multiple sclerosis

B12 helps lower homocysteine levels, which is important as homocysteine has been linked to an increased risk of heart disease.

Deficiencies in B12 can lead to:

- Dementia
- Neuropathy
- Liver illnesses and disease
- Neuropathy
- Demyelination of the brain
- Sore tongue
- Pernicious Anemia
- Diarrhea

Chapter 23
Vitamin C

Vitamin C might be the most important of all the vitamins, as it is necessary for and helps with many bodily functions.

About 2 million sailors were killed by scurvy between the 16th and 18th centuries. Often, half of the crew could die on a long voyage in the sea.

In the mid-1700s, the British physician James Lind ran an experiment and discovered that sailors who ate oranges and lemons were able to lessen and get rid of the effects of scurvy. The thing in the oranges and lemons that helped treat scurvy was later discovered to be Vitamin C.

According to the CDC, 10% to 17% of low-income Americans have low vitamin C levels that can cause full-blown scurvy. Eighty-two of people with severe COVID had extremely low vitamin C levels, according to the Nutrition Journal in 2021.

Most animals can make vitamin C, and they create a whole lot more when they get under stress. Humans are one of the few animals that can't make their own vitamin C, along with many primates, guinea pigs, fruit bats, and capybaras. Thus, humans need to get Vitamin C from their diets and by supplementing.

Heavy smoking of cigarettes daily leads to lower reserves of Vitamin C.

Vitamin C can also help with blood sugar issues.

Vitamin C helps with heart health and lowers your risk of heart disease. Animals that make their own vitamin C generally do not suffer coronary heart attacks. When it actually does occur, it is extremely rare and correlated to a deficiency in Vitamin C. Dr. Matthias Rath discusses this in his book Why Animals Don't Get Heart Attacks But Humans Do. Dr. Rath writes, "Why animals don't get heart attacks, but every second man and woman die from them: Animals don't get heart attacks because they produce large amounts of vitamin C in their bodies. Vitamin C optimizes the production of collagen and other reinforcement molecules, thereby stabilizing the walls of the arteries and preventing atherosclerotic deposits, heart attacks, and strokes. We human beings cannot manufacture a single molecule of vitamin C in our bodies, and almost everyone gets too few vitamins from their diet. The inevitable consequence of this is a weakening of the artery wall deposits (atherosclerosis)."

Vitamin C can be found in citrus fruits (e.g., oranges and lemons), dark leafy green vegetables, strawberries, potatoes, tomatoes, peppers (green, red, and yellow), broccoli, brussel sprouts, kale, guava, papaya, and kiwi.

Vitamin C is water-soluble. As an antioxidant, it protects cholesterol and cells from oxidative damage.

Vitamin C can increase the red blood cell levels of the very important antioxidant glutathione.

Vitamin C helps regenerate Vitamin E in the body from its oxidized form.

Vitamin C is a histamine scavenger, and one molecule of vitamin C destroys another molecule of histamine. The big buildup of histamine in the body is the main cause of the loosening of collagen fibers and bleeding tissues in the scurvy. The collagen fibers and tissues don't have enough Vitamin C.

Vitamin C is also extremely important for the ability of the liver to detoxify substances in the body. Vitamin C does this through its antioxidant actions by raising glutathione levels.

Vitamin C also reduces the risk of heart disease. It also prevents the oxidation of cholesterol, which many consider a factor in atherosclerosis.

Vitamin C is necessary to produce collagen. Collagen is a protein that makes the connective tissue that helps hold our skin intact. Collagen is also a very vital constituent of blood vessels, tendons, cartilage, and ligaments.

Vitamin C also makes the capillaries stronger. This can help people recover from bruises faster.

Vitamin C is concentrated in white blood cells, which are very important parts of the immune system as they protect against and fight infection.

Vitamin C helps boost the levels of interferon. Interferon is an antiviral chemical that your body produces that is necessary to make protective hormones. Interferon is also needed to help battle against cancer.

It is best to take Vitamin C in divided doses throughout the day.

Vitamin C helps with arthritis because of its anti-inflammatory properties.

Vitamin C helps reduce the risk of getting peripheral artery disease and atherosclerosis.

Vitamin C can help reduce the allergic response in people with asthma. It can also reduce the risk of respiratory tract infections for people with asthma.

One study had people with asthma take 1,000 mg of Vitamin C for 14 weeks; another group took a placebo. After 14 weeks, the group that took Vitamin C had 73% fewer asthma attacks than those in the placebo group. The attacks were also less severe in the Vitamin C group.

Vitamin C can help fight against cancer by supporting the proper operation of the immune and white blood cells.

Vitamin C can help prevent cataracts from forming by preventing oxidation in the lens of the eye. Oxidation plays a major part in cataract formation.

Numerous studies have shown that Vitamin C reduces both the severity and length of colds.

People with diabetes usually have a Vitamin C deficiency, so it is a good idea to boost your dosage of Vitamin C if you have diabetes.

Research also shows that Vitamin C can help reduce wrinkles.

Vitamin C has been shown to have antiviral and antibiotic properties.

Vitamin C also helps reduce some of the harmful effects of ultraviolet rays of the sun.

If you suffer from gingivitis and have bleeding gums and gum inflammation, you might have a Vitamin C deficiency.

People who suffer from glaucoma have increased pressure within their eyeballs. Vitamin C has been shown to help reduce that pressure.

More research has been coming out demonstrating that Vitamin C lessens your risk of getting gallstones. Vitamin C does this by triggering an enzyme that breaks down cholesterol into bile acids. This is crucial because gallstones appear when the blood becomes very saturated with cholesterol.

Vitamin C can help with hepatitis because it activates the white blood cells of the immune system, and that aids in keeping the hepatitis virus under control.

Vitamin C helps with male infertility. One study done in infertile men demonstrated that 1,000 mg supplements two times a day for two months increased sperm count by more than 100% and boosted sperm motility by 92%. Deformed sperm was decreased by 55%.

Vitamin C helps reduce the risk of heart disease. It prevents the oxidation of lipoproteins and LDL cholesterol, which often are precursors of hardening of the arteries (atherosclerosis). It also raises what is called the good cholesterol (LDL cholesterol).

High levels of Vitamin C are linked with lower blood pressure. Blood pressure is a risk factor for cardiovascular disease. So, if you can lower blood pressure, that is good for your heart. Vitamin C fortifies and strengthens the collagen in the artery walls. That leads to the artery walls becoming stronger and less susceptible to scarring.

Vitamin C is very important for helping you to deal with stress. Vitamin C is involved in the formation of stress hormones by the adrenal glands, which are the stress glands. Stress is known to deplete you of Vitamin C, so taking an abundance of Vitamin C is important, especially if you get stressed often.

Notably, a study published in Nutrients showed that increasing your Vitamin C intake may significantly decrease the risk of cardiovascular mortality (CVM).

In the Seguimiento Universidad de Navarra (SUN) project, over the course of 11 years, they collected data from 13,421 individuals. They mailed questionnaires to participants every two years to get the data from them. They were asked to disclose how often they had eaten and drunk 136 different foods and beverages in the past 12 months. This would allow the researchers to comprehend not just the Vitamin C levels in the participants' diets but other variables like calorie intake and fiber. The participants were also required to provide the researchers with all medical details on any cardiovascular events they went through during this time. They discovered from the analyzed data that those with a higher intake of Vitamin C were 70% less likely to suffer from cardiovascular mortality than those with a lower intake.

Vitamin C can help prevent gout and reduce uric acid levels in the blood. Gout is a form of arthritis that affects approximately 4% of adults in the United States and causes severe pain, swelling, redness, and tenderness in joints. High levels of uric acid can cause a whole bunch of health issues, including heart disease, kidney disease, diabetes, fatty liver disease, and high blood pressure. High uric acid can also damage your bones, joints, tendons, and ligaments.

One study followed 46,994 healthy men over 20 years to see if there was a link between taking Vitamin C and developing gout. The study concluded that men who supplement with Vitamin C had a lowered risk of developing gout by 44%.

An analysis of 13 studies discovered that taking a vitamin C supplement for 30 days greatly decreased blood uric acid compared with a placebo.

Vitamin C can help protect your thinking and memory as you get older. Vitamin C is required to develop, grow, and repair all body tissues. You also need Vitamin C to maintain teeth, bones, and cartilage. Vitamin C can also help slow down Age-Related Macular Degeneration.

Vitamin C can also help speed healing.

People who eat diets high in vitamin C tend to be less frequently diagnosed with arthritis.

Vitamin C is the most important nutrient for the adrenal gland. Vitamin C helps with iron absorption. It helps with wound repair. Vitamin C may help prevent certain types of cancer. It will boost immunity. Vitamin C will help shield against sun damage. It will also protect you from free radical damage. Vitamin C supports brain health.

Vitamin C may help lower blood pressure. An analysis of 29 studies on humans discovered that taking a vitamin C supplement lowered systolic blood pressure (the upper number) by 3.8 mmHg and diastolic blood pressure (the lower number) by 1.5 mmHg on average in adults.

Vitamin C may be the master vitamin. Vitamin C is an antioxidant that is involved in numerous bodily functions. It requires the repair of all body tissues and for growth and development. Vitamin C helps build collagen and aids in supporting a healthy immune system.

One of the forms of Vitamin C is ascorbic acid. "A" in chemistry means without. "Scorbic" means scurvy. So ascorbic means without scurvy.

Vitamin C is very crucial in the synthesis of connective tissue. Vitamin C is very important for your bones. Bones require collagen, and you need Vitamin C to build collagen.

Vitamin C is very important for your skin and antiaging.

Humans are one of the living beings who can't make their own vitamin C, along with primates and guinea pigs. All other animals can make vitamin C, and when an animal is under stress, it makes vitamin C.

Signs of Vitamin C deficiency include:

- Bleeding Gums
- Scurvy
- Increase Cancer Risk
- Dry and Rough skin
- Easy Bruising
- Swollen and Painful Joints
- Slow Healing of Wounds
- Weak Bones
- Depressed Immune System
- Fatigue
- Poor Growth
- Loose Teeth

Food Sources of Vitamin C include:

- Citrus Fruits (e.g., oranges and lemons)
- Dark, Leafy Green Vegetables
- Strawberries
- Potatoes
- Tomatoes
- Peppers (Green, Red, and Yellow)
- Broccoli
- Brussel Sprouts
- Kale
- Papaya
- Kiwi
- Guava

Chapter 24
Vitamin D

Vitamin D is known as the Sunshine Vitamin because the best source of Vitamin D is the sun. Vitamin D is one of the fat-soluble vitamins (A, D, E, and K). Fat-soluble means it is stored within the liver and other fatty tissues when not used. When the body needs them, then they are secreted.

Vitamin D is actually a steroid hormone. It is similar to testosterone.

The best source of Vitamin D is the sun. Daily sunshine exposure of 20-30 minutes per day is recommended to get your Vitamin D, especially on your arms or legs.

Vitamin D is awesome for your immunity. People get sick more frequently during the winter because they are not in the sun much because it is cold. And even when they go out in the sun, they have most of their body covered, so they can't get much of the vitamin D from the sun.

When you have optimal levels of Vitamin D, it has been shown to help the immune system effectively ward off pathogens.

Vitamin D can help keep the teeth and bones strong. Vitamin D can also fight diseases such as heart disease, cancer, and neurodegenerative conditions.

Vitamin D supplementation reduces autoimmune diseases by 22%, according to a study published in the BMJ in 2022.

Those infected with the Wuhan coronavirus (COVID-19) had a lower death risk when given vitamin D along with the standard treatment, according to a study published in January 2021 in the journal Current Opinion in Clinical Nutrition and Metabolic Care. The authors of the study also added that the COVID-19 mortality risk was lowered by about 60 percent if vitamin D was given early enough.

Vitamin D was shown to be able to both treat and prevent SARS in 2003.

Because Vitamin D can help detoxify carcinogenic heavy metals, which makes it a critical cancer-fighting vitamin. Vitamin D3 also causes cellular differentiation (the opposite of cancer) when it is activated in the kidneys and liver. Vitamin D can inhibit the growth of malignant cancer cells. It can also prevent the development of new blood vessels that supply nutrients and carry the malignant cells throughout the body.

Vitamin D deficiency is common in the United States. This has resulted in increased susceptibility to various health issues and problems. Vitamin D deficiency has been linked to dementia and Alzheimer's disease. Other conditions that occur as a result of Vitamin D deficiency include respiratory infections, depression, and multiple sclerosis.

Some foods contain Vitamin D, but supplementation is often required to get ideal levels in the blood.

To get the maximum benefits of Vitamin D, it is recommended you take Vitamin D3 (cholecalciferol). Vitamin D2 (ergocalciferol), which comes from plants, won't give you the same number of benefits as Vitamin D3.

Vitamin D can help strengthen bones. A study published in Nutrients in 2010 stated that over long periods of time, inadequate Vitamin D intake can lead to bone demineralization, which is when you lose minerals in the bone quicker than you can replace those minerals. Bone demineralization has been linked to different conditions, such as osteomalacia (bone softening), osteoporosis (severe bone brittleness and weakness) in adults, and rickets in children.

Vitamin D has also been linked to improved outcomes in dealing with cancer. The sunshine vitamin has been known to suppress cancer growth and the formation of blood vessels that feed the cancer cells in colon, prostate, and breast cancer.

A breast cancer study showed that 24 percent in the breast cancer study had adequate levels of vitamin D at the time of diagnosis. People who were deficient in Vitamin D were more likely to have the cancer return years later or metastasize or recur ten years later. Seventy-three percent of those who were Vitamin D deficient were more likely to die.

It was discovered in a study in the journal International Journal of Cancer that vitamin D protects cells from oxidative stress. It helps relieve cell stress and retains healthy cells.

If you want to lose some weight, you may want to consider raising your levels of Vitamin D3 either through diet or by sunlight exposure. Studies have shown that increasing your vitamin D level by getting out in the sun, eating more foods with Vitamin D or taking a Vitamin D3 supplement combined with exercising and eating a good and nutritious diet can help you lose weight. One reason this happens is because Vitamin D3 helps to keep your body fat levels down. Research has also shown that people deficient in Vitamin D have a higher risk of becoming obese.

Rheumatoid arthritis is a chronic inflammatory disease of the joints. Studies have shown that people with rheumatoid arthritis often have low levels of Vitamin D. Rheumatoid arthritis is an autoimmune disease. Inflammation in the joints is caused by your immune system acting as if the proteins in the lining of the joints are enemy invaders and foreign substances. The immune system reacts to the linings of the joints as if these proteins were foreign substances. The inflammation results in pain, reduced mobility and stiffness, deformed joints, and bone loss.

Now, since one of the main benefits of vitamin D is that it helps the immune system function properly, it makes sense that a vitamin D deficiency could lead to health problems and immune system issues. It is a good idea to increase your Vitamin D dosage to help with rheumatoid arthritis.

Several long-term studies have shown an association between low Vitamin D levels and high blood pressure (high blood pressure). Thus, higher levels of Vitamin D can help lower blood pressure. If you suffer from high blood pressure or want to avoid getting it, raising your Vitamin D levels can help.

There are more and more studies showing that Vitamin D deficiency is a risk factor for developing heart disease, congestive heart failure, heart attacks, strokes, and peripheral arterial disease. Increasing your Vitamin D levels can help lower the risk of developing heart disease.

Vitamin D helps improve your daily mood, especially in the colder, darker months. People tend to feel more down and depressed during the month. Some studies have shown that the symptoms of Seasonal Affective Disorder (SAD) could be linked to low levels of Vitamin D3 due to the lack of sunlight exposure during the cold and dark winter months. SAD is a mood disorder whose main symptom is depression. Since people are not out in the sun much during the winter and are not getting Vitamin D from the sun, that is probably one of the reasons why people feel more down and depressed during the winter since they are not out in the sun much.

Various studies suggest that the levels of Vitamin D3 may impact the levels of serotonin in the body. Serotonin is a hormone that regulates mood. Raising your Vitamin D3 level can raise the level of serotonin in your body, which in turn can boost your mood.

Most people in the United States and Western societies are familiar with or have heard of diabetes, particularly type II diabetes. Since most people with diabetes have Type II diabetes, this is the one that is more highly publicized. Recent research has shown that people who get big amounts of vitamin D as children have a reduced risk of developing type I diabetes later on in life.

Type I diabetes is not the same but different from type II diabetes in that type I does not arise out of insulin resistance; Type I happens as a result of the insulin-producing beta cells in the pancreas being ravaged by the person's own immune system, beginning early in childhood.

A 2018 study in the Journal of the Academy of Orthopaedic Surgeons said that Vitamin D is influential in strengthening the muscle. According to Lana Nasrallah, MPH, RD, clinical dietician at UNC Health, "Lack of vitamin D in the body can increase the risk of having weak muscles, which in turn increases the risk of falls." Nasrallah also says, "Vitamin D may help increase muscle strength, thus preventing falls, which is a common problem that leads to substantial disability and death in older adults."

Chapter 25
Vitamin E

Vitamin E is a natural blood thinner. Hospitals know that since they often will tell you not to take any Vitamin E either right before or after an operation since it can cause bleeding. Yet when they prescribe a blood thinner, doctors almost never prescribe Vitamin E. They will describe things like warfarin, which is made from rat poison.

The two most common forms of Vitamin E are the tocopherols and the tocotrienols.

Vitamin E has many benefits.

Vitmain E aids in the production of collagen. It also helps with acne. Vitamin E helps with AIDS. People with AIDS are usually deficient in vitamin E. Taking vitamin E helps slow down the progression of AIDS.

Vitamin E, working together with selenium, can help lower the risk of certain cancers.

Vitamin E helps reduce the risk of dementia and Alzheimer's disease.

Vitamin E also helps protect against heart disease and strokes. It can also help prevent and treat angina.

Vitamin E has a natural anti-inflammatory effect and can help people who suffer from various forms of arthritis, especially rheumatoid arthritis.

Cataracts happen because of the oxidation that happens to the lens of the eye. The antioxidant vitamin E can help prevent cataracts.

Vitamin E can help prevent macular degeneration of the eye and can help improve the condition.

Vitamin E also helps protect against heart disease and strokes. It can also help prevent and treat angina.

Vitamin E helps lessen hot flashes and vaginal dryness in women going through menopause. Vitamin E helps with the immune system. Vitamin E can help reduce eczema. Vitamin E increases HDL levels and prevents the oxidation of cholesterol.

Vitamin E helps with male fertility. In fact, one of the forms of Vitamin E, tocopherol, comes from the Greek word "to bear young" or "to bear children."

Studies demonstrate that persons with low levels of Vitamin E tend to be more susceptible to various forms of cancer. Vitamin E can help prevent some cancers, particularly lung and prostate cancer.

Vitamin E also promotes the healing of wounds to the skin and burns. Vitamin E improves glucose tolerance in people with diabetes. It also helps shield against nerve damage that is associated with free radical damage brought about by diabetes.

Deficiencies in Vitamin E can lead to:

- Fertility Problems
- Alzheimer's Diseases
- Depressed Immune System
- Anemia
- Increased Risk of Cancer
- Difficulty Walking
- Muscle Weakness or Pain
- Numbness and Tingling
- Deterioration in Vision

Chapter 26
Vitamin K

Vitamin K is a fat-soluble vitamin like Vitamins A, D, and E. It is stored in the fat tissue and the liver.

Vitamin K comes in two forms. The first form is called phylloquinone (Vitamin K1) and has one molecule. This is found in green leafy vegetables like cabbage, lettuce, collard greens, kale, and spinach. The second is called menaquinone (Vitamin K2) and has multiple molecules. Menaquinones are found in fermented foods such as the Japanese natto, beef liver, chicken, eel, and sauerkraut. Cheese and eggs may have small amounts. They are also produced by bacteria in the human body.

Vitamin K is necessary to help make various proteins that are required for the clotting of blood and for the building of bones. Prothrombin is made by the liver and is a vitamin K-dependent protein directly involved with blood clotting. Prothrombin is converted into thrombin in the clotting of blood. Another protein that needs vitamin K to produce strong, healthy bone tissue is osteocalcin.

Vitamin K can be found throughout the body, including the brain, heart, bone, liver, and pancreas. Vitamin K rarely reaches dangerous and toxic levels in the body because it breaks down very quickly and is excreted in the stool or urine.

Vitamin K supports the blood clotting process. Vitamin K2 is a major calcium-processing substance. Vitamin K2 keeps calcium in the bones, keeps calcium out of the blood, and helps prevent calcification. Vitamin K2 also improves arterial flexibility.

Vitamin K2 helps with bone formation and repair.

Getting enough Vitamin K2 has been linked to a decreased risk of heart disease and hip fractures.

The Rotterdam study looked at Vitamin K2. It looked at 4,807 healthy people who were 55 and older. The results suggested a higher dietary intake of Vitamin K2 had a strong protective effect on arterial calcification. The study showed a decrease of as much as 50 percent in cardiovascular diseases and deaths related to cardiovascular disease for those who took more Vitamin K2. Also, the all-cause mortality rate was reduced by 25 percent for individuals who took high amounts of Vitamin K2.

In a 3-year, double-blind study, 22 healthy postmenopausal Dutch women were randomly given Vitamin K2 in its MK-7 form or placebo capsules. The results showed that the women given Vitamin K2 showed marked improvement in arterial stiffness. That is, arterial elasticity was improved compared to that of those given the placebo.

Another study that appeared in the journal Nutrition, Metabolism and Cardiovascular Diseases looked at the effect of Vitamin K2 on the ability to relax and contract blood vessels. They followed 16,057 women who were free of any type of cardiovascular illness for eight years. They found that Vitamin K2 reduced the risk of cardiovascular diseases. Coronary heart disease risk decreased by 9 percent for every 10 micrograms of Vitamin K2 the participants ingested.

Vitamin K is an essential nutrient. You can't live without it. Vitamin K helps with osteoporosis.

In cases of Vitamin K deficiency, calcium that is free usually goes looking for a place to go to and often goes to the arteries. That can cause the arteries to stiffen, and harmful blood clots can form. Vitamin K helps defend against dangerous calcification of the arteries.

Our bone builders are called osteoblasts. The osteoblasts make a protein called osteocalcin. Osteocalcin needs to first be activated by Vitamin K2 in order to be able to properly bind calcium to the bones. Calcium is very important to maintain bone strength and prevent fractures and osteoporosis. Vitamin K2 turns on the light switch. If you don't have Vitamin K2, you won't be able to activate osteocalcin, which takes the calcium to where it is needed. It will also keep that calcium there.

People who have hip fractures tend to have low levels of Vitamin K. Natto is the richest source of Vitamin K2 in MK-7 form. People who consumed high levels of natto had reduced risks of fractures, according to a 2001 study in the journal Nutrition. A clinical study from 2006 covered 944 women from ages 20 to 79. That study showed that consuming natto led to inhibiting loss of bone mineral density.

Vitamin K2 from natto was featured in a 2008 study in the Journal of Epidemiology as a vital part of improved bone health. The consumption of K2 strongly correlated with decreasing the risk of hip fractures.

Vitamin K deficiencies can lead to:

- Osteoarthritis
- Liver disease
- Weakened Bones
- Increased Clotting Time
- Nose Bleeds
- Osteoporosis
- Calcium not being properly absorbed as well as not being properly deposited in the bones.

Make sure to get enough Vitamin K in your diet.

Chapter 27
Calcium

Calcium is a very important mineral. Calcium makes up 2% of your body weight, which is more than any other mineral.

You want calcium in your bones and not in your arteries.

Calcium has numerous benefits. Calcium helps with the symptoms of P.M.S. Calcium is a factor in sperm motility and enzyme reactions. It helps your heartbeat, helps your hormones stay active, helps set up the release of neurotransmitters, smooths the path for cell division, helps contract your muscles, and helps to keep your nerves lively.

If you use calcium supplements, use those that also contain magnesium. Magnesium helps you absorb calcium better, and magnesium offsets the action of calcium, allowing you to avoid calcification.

At least 147 different diseases can be attributed to either a deficiency in calcium or an imbalance.

If you lack stomach acid or Vitamin D, you will likely develop a calcium deficiency. Calcium plays a key role in blood clotting. Some studies suggest calcium may help reduce the risk of colon cancer.

Calcium is required to build strong teeth and for good dental health. Tooth development in children is supported by calcium. Calcium strengthens the enamel of the teeth, which helps protect our teeth from erosion, decay, and cavities.

Calcium helps with hyperparathyroidism (or overactive parathyroid). Taking calcium orally decreases parathyroid hormone levels in people with high parathyroid hormone levels.

Several studies indicate that people with low calcium levels are more likely to gain weight. Calcium is involved in maintaining a healthy metabolism, which is required to maintain a healthy weight. Calcium may also help lower blood pressure.

Calcium may help with a lower risk of colorectal adenomas, which is a type of non-cancerous tumor. Consuming calcium during pregnancy can help in lowering blood pressure and reduce the risk of preeclampsia.

Calcium is a cofactor for many enzymes; some important enzymes cannot work efficiently without calcium.

Calcium deficiencies lead to many diseases, such as osteoporosis and Bell's Palsy. Up to 147 diseases may be attributed to a calcium deficiency.

Many people think kidney stones come from too much calcium. It actually comes from too little calcium. When you have a calcium deficiency, your body leeches calcium from your bones. Take more calcium to prevent kidney stones. Calcium helps with building strong bones.

Sources of Calcium include:

1. Dairy
2. Cheese
3. Almonds
4. Sardines
5. Seeds
6. Leafy greens
7. Edamame
8. White Beans
9. Whey Protein
10. Figs
11. Legumes
12. Cornmeal
13. Black Beans

The bones store calcium and need high calcium levels to stay strong. When you become deficient and have low levels of calcium, the body often diverts some of the calcium from the bones, which makes them more brittle and prone to injury.

Having low levels of calcium can lead to osteopenia, which is a decrease in mineral density in the bones. This can eventually lead to osteoporosis. Osteoporosis causes the bones to become thin and brittle and vulnerable to fractures, as well as problems with posture and pain.

Severe premenstrual syndrome (PMS) has been associated with low levels of calcium. A 2017 study found that participants reported lower rates of fluid retention and improved mood after two months of taking 500 milligrams (mg) of calcium daily.

When the body becomes deficient in calcium, it starts leeching it from sources such as the teeth. This can eventually cause dental issues like brittle teeth, tooth decay, and irritated gums. Lack of calcium can hurt tooth development in infants.

Symptoms of Calcium Deficiency include:

- Receding Gums
- Brittle teeth
- Muscle aches, spasms and cramps
- Depression
- Numbness
- Fatigue
- Kidney Stones
- Arthritis
- Osteoporosis
- Confusion
- Hallucinations
- Twitching or tremors
- Weak and brittle nails
- Easy bone fractures
- Arrhythmias
- Bell's Palsy
- Tinnitus (Ringing in the ears)
- Low Back Pain
- Elevated Blood Pressure
- Poor Clotting
- Dry skin
- Coarse hair
- Alopecia
- Eczema
- Psoriasis
- Pain in the arms and thighs when walking or moving
- Cataracts
- Insomnia

Chapter 28
Copper

Copper is another important mineral that people are deficient in. Aneurysms have been linked to copper deficiencies. Grey hair has also been linked to a deficiency of copper. Copper helps with varicose veins.

Copper is important for several functions, including:

- Absorption of iron
- Helping with the immune system
- Production of red blood cells
- Development of organs like the heart and the brain
- Development, maintenance, and sustenance of bones and connective tissue
- Prevention of the inflammation of the prostate
- Helps with the formation of collagen
- Helps regulate heart rate and blood pressure
- Helps with energy levels
- Helps with brain function
- Helps with skin and hair health
- Reduces inflammation
- Aids in maintaining the strength of connective tissue and organs
- Helps with thyroid health, neurological health, heart health, and arthritis

Make sure you get enough copper, and supplement if necessary.

Food sources of iron include:

- Almonds
- Avocado
- Beef Liver
- Oysters
- Potatoes
- Salmon
- Kale
- Spinach

- Dark Chocolate
- Turnip Greens
- Kale
- Chia Seeds
- Cashews
- Sesame Seeds
- Salmon

Chapter 29
Iodine

Iodine is another great mineral for your health.

Low levels of iodine in more than 50% of the population have been indicated in the National Health and Nutrition Examination Survey studies.

Physicians used to routinely use iodine in their medical practice. The typical dose used by doctors was 1 gram of potassium iodide that contained 770 mg of iodine. That was much greater than the U.S. RDA of 150 mcg.

Iodine is mostly known for proper thyroid function and proper metabolisms. Iodine is also important to have a healthy immune system.

Iodine also has antiviral, anticancer, antibacterial, and antiparasitic properties.

The main storage site for iodine in the body is the thyroid. You can also find iodine in the glandular system, including the sweat glands. High concentrations of iodine are found in the brain, ovaries, breasts, and prostate. Just about every cell in the body is dependent on iodine. When you are deficient in iodine, the thyroid will compete with other storage areas for it. All of the storage sites will eventually become depleted. This depletion puts you at risk for a whole bunch of illnesses, including cancer.

Children's growth and development is dependent on iodine. According to the World Health Organization, Iodine deficiency in pregnant women is the primary cause of brain damage and mental retardation.

Your body needs a certain amount of iodine every day for your thyroid to work normally, as it plays an extremely important role in the healthy function of your thyroid.

One of the key roles and functions of the thyroid gland is metabolism. As iodine is vital for healthy thyroid function, supplementing it with iodine can support a healthy metabolism.

Iodine helps maintain healthy energy levels. Iodine plays a very important role in the conversion of food into energy and in the effective use of calories. Among iodine-deficient people, iodine intake is associated with improved energy levels.

If you want healthy and glowing skin, getting enough iodine in your diet is important. Iodine also supports healthy hair growth.

Iodine can help improve your immunity by promoting antioxidant activity in your body. It will also protect your cells from oxidative stress.

The thyroid requires iodine to produce its hormones and to regulate the body's metabolism. Hypothyroidism is marked by a low metabolic rate. Hypothyroidism has some of the following systems: fatigue, not being able to concentrate, muscle cramps, muscle weakness, weight gain, brittle nails, infertility, dry skin, cold hands and feet, and puffy eyes. When people are iodine deficient, then hypothyroidism becomes more common. Supplementing with iodine often results in improving or even curing the hypothyroid condition. Chronic deficiencies in iodine and the body not being able to properly make use of iodine paves the way for cancers of hormone-sensitive tissues and glands, like the prostate, uterus, ovaries, and breasts.

Iodine was replaced by bromine in the 1980s as an ingredient in bread dough. Unfortunately, bromine is known as a carcinogen. This has led to an increase in bromide toxicity and increases in thyroid cancer, thyroid disorders, and various other illnesses resulting from this iodine deficiency as a result of being taken out of the bread doughs. Bromine is also used in pest control, in some prescription medications, crop fumigation, pest control, and in some carbonated drinks.

The body does not produce iodine. It is also not easy to get adequate iodine from the diet. There is a great amount in the ocean. The soil around the oceans usually has enough iodine. Sea vegetables (seaweed) are a good source of iodine. Fish also contain iodine. Inland and mountainous areas have little iodine. The detoxifying effect of iodine also bolsters the immune system and helps balance hormones.

Getting sufficient iodine supplementation helps treat many conditions, including thyroid disorders, infertility, vaginal infections, attention deficit disorder, sebaceous cysts, prostate, ovarian and breast diseases (including cancer), and many others.

Sufficient amounts of iodine are critical for pregnant women both for their well-being and the healthy development of their babies. Iodine deficiencies during pregnancy can have severe consequences for both mother and baby.

Some people think iodine supplementation causes goiter. It is actually an iodine deficiency that causes goiter.

Iodine deficiency has been linked as a cause of breast cancer. A higher incidence of breast cancer has been found in iodine-deficient areas. Iodine and thyroid hormones often reduce the risk of breast cancer.

Japan has a low rate of breast cancer, and some researchers believe that is because of the iodine-rich diet.

Breast milk has a greater amount of iodine than does formula milk. Formula-fed premature babies may also be at risk of deficiency in iodine. Some good sources of iodine include seaweed, kelp, onions, dairy, saltwater fish, seafood, and beans.

The second highest concentration of iodine (after the thyroid) is found in women's breast tissue. The risk of acquiring breast cancer is increased when the iodine level is reduced. Also, women who get breast cancer usually have higher levels of estrogen and lower levels of progesterone in the breast tissue. Progesterone helps keep estrogen levels in check.

Iodine is used to detoxify lead, aluminum, and mercury. Iodine helps shrink cysts in the thyroid, uterus, ovaries, and breast. Iodine aids in regulating estrogen dominance. Iodine helps slash the size of skin tags and warts. Iodine helps against cancer. Iodine aids with scar regeneration.

Iodine can help boost your mood. Iodine helps reduce stones in the parotid gland. The parotid gland makes saliva.

Since it balances estrogen, iodine can help lessen hot flashes and reduce cystic acne.

Chapter 30
Iron

Iron is another important mineral that your body needs for development and growth. Iron is necessary for red blood cell production. It is used by your body to make hemoglobin, a protein in red blood cells that carries oxygen from the lungs to all body parts. Your body also uses iron to make myoglobin, which is a protein that provides oxygen to the muscles. Iron is also needed to make some hormones.

Iron helps fortify the immune system, enhances sleep quality, and provides support for pregnant women. It also helps prevent anemia and promotes fetal health. Iron is vital for healthy brain development and growth in children. Vitamin C enhances the absorption of iron.

Iron also helps with skin nourishment and the reduction of dark circles. It also helps with enhanced memory, hair health, and enhanced sports performance. Other benefits of iron include reduced fatigue and enhanced concentration.

There are two types of dietary iron. They are heme and non-heme. Heme iron can be found in animal food sources, including meat and seafood. The body more easily absorbs heme iron than non-heme iron. Heme iron's bioavailability from animal sources can be up to 40 percent.

On the other hand, non-heme iron, found in plants, requires the body to take several steps to absorb it. Plant-based sources of iron include fortified grain, vegetables, beans, nuts, and soy.

Non-heme iron from plant-based sources has a bioavailability of between 2 and 20%, which is significantly less than for heme iron. That is why the RDA for vegetarians is 1.8 times higher than those who eat meat to compensate for lower absorption levels from plant-based food.

Taking non-heme iron sources alongside foods that are rich in Vitamin C can greatly increase iron absorption.

Iron deficiency anemia often occurs in individuals who lose blood or do not consume animal products. Symptoms of iron deficiency anemia include fatigue/tiredness, weakness, lower energy, weakened immunity, lack of concentration, learning disabilities in children, digestive problems, cognitive issues, and temperature regulation difficulties.

Food sources of iron include:

- Eggs
- Organ meats like live
- Poultry meat
- Red meat
- Fish such as sardines, tuna, and salmon
- Beans, lentils, peas
- Tofu
- Shellfish
- Spinach, kale and broccoli
- Nuts

One thing to be aware of is that even though it is very important to have enough iron in your diet, very high levels of iron can be dangerous to your health. Elevated levels of iron can harm your joints, tissues, and organs. They also raise your risk of diabetes, heart disease, cancer, obesity, and early death, among other diseases.

Women excrete about 500 ml of iron every year through menstruation. Women shed iron every month for about 30 years, so women generally have a longer life expectancy than men. Men are not able to regularly excrete large amounts of iron. As a result, men have consistently higher levels of iron than premenopausal women.

Once women hit menopause, they also lose the ability to excrete significant amounts of iron.

As you get older, checking your iron levels is more important. One thing you can do to lower your iron levels is to donate blood. While reducing your iron donating blood, you will also help other people at the same time.

Which People Need Iron Supplements?

These people might require iron supplements:
1) Babies, especially low birth weight or premature babies
2) Women during menstruation (they need twice as much iron as men do)
3) People who donate blood frequently
4) Pregnant women
5) People with iron deficiency anemia

Chapter 31
Magnesium

Your body needs different vitamins and minerals to function properly. One incredibly important mineral is magnesium, which acts as fuel for your busy body. Magnesium is often called the Master Mineral. You will have many problems and issues with various bodily functions if you are deficient in magnesium. Magnesium aids and supports many physiological processes, including sleep and relaxation.

65% of people admitted to the ICU (Intensive Care Unit) are deficient in magnesium. If you want to stay out of and avoid the ICU, then make sure you are getting enough magnesium. Phosphoric acid drains magnesium. Stress, antibiotics, and diuretics also lower magnesium.

Obtaining an adequate amount of magnesium helps ensure that you will have a healthy heart, skeletal system, and inflammatory response. Magnesium also helps support blood sugar and energy levels and helps maintain steady blood pressure.

Magnesium fuels more than 800 enzyme processes in your body, according to magnesium authority Dr. Carolyn Dean. It is extremely deficient in the soil as well as in the food supply, so you will need to take supplements to get your required daily amounts of magnesium.

While doctors prescribe all kinds of calcium channel-blocking drugs, magnesium is the ultimate calcium channel blocker without the side effects.

Long-term stress will increase the stress hormone adrenaline, which will decrease your magnesium levels.

These things will decrease magnesium levels:

1. Pharmaceutical drugs.
2. Fluoride and fluorine in the water.
3. Food processing.
4. Herbicides and pesticides.
5. Caffeine will deplete magnesium because of its diuretic effect.
6. Working out, athletic performance, and exercising will cause loss of magnesium through sweating.

7. Alcohol will deplete magnesium because of the diuretic effect.
8. Magnesium absorption is decreased by antacids and heartburn drugs that decrease stomach acid.
9. Junk foods, especially sugar products, deplete magnesium.
10. Stress and trauma can decrease magnesium levels.
11. Refining grains reduces magnesium.
12. Taking statin drugs.
13. Insulin.

Many drug side effects turn out to be magnesium deficiency symptoms, as many drugs deplete the body of magnesium.
If you drink soda and soft drinks, you can become magnesium deficient because sugar uses up magnesium.
Production of cortisol and norepinephrine can cause your body to become depleted of magnesium.
Even a small magnesium deficiency can cause a person to become hyperexcitable, according to a 2015 study. This is shown in the EEG measurements. Magnesium will slow down your heart response to sleep problems, exercise, and sympathetic nervous system stimulation.
Magnesium sulfate may relieve restless legs syndrome in pregnancy.
Coffee, sugar, smoking, and alcohol can deplete magnesium.
Magnesium relaxes the tension in the neck and head that make migraines worse. Magnesium will help balance blood sugar.
Magnesium has little or no tendency to interact with medical drugs people take.
Magnesium helps prevent spasms in the artery as well as prevent the formation of blood clots.
Many people know that nitric oxide controls vasodilation, but many people are unaware that this activity is under the direction of magnesium.
Magnesium is kept in emergency rooms for heart attack patients.
Magnesium can aid in clearing pollution in your lungs and can help prevent bronchial spasms.
There will be no calcification of body parts unless you have too little magnesium to keep the calcium in balance.
Calcification can be initiated by inflammation. A major cause of inflammation in the human body is having a magnesium deficiency with an excess of calcium.

Calcium channel blockers deplete magnesium. Diuretics drain the body of magnesium even more. As these drugs drain the body of magnesium, it makes people susceptible to atrial fibrillation. Muscle twitches and spasms are signs of magnesium deficiency. Magnesium will help release those spasms. Magnesium helps with muscle cramps and lower back pain.

Magnesium aids your body to utilize, absorb, and digest fats, carbohydrates, and proteins. Magnesium is required for insulin to open the cell membranes for glucose entry. Magnesium will also help block obesity genes from expressing themselves. People who suffer from diabetes lose more magnesium than most people and require more magnesium as their magnesium levels are low. Magnesium is required for the transport, operation, and production of insulin. The main function of insulin requires magnesium, and insulin won't be properly secreted from the pancreas without magnesium. Whatever does get into the bloodstream won't function correctly. Magnesium is also a vital cofactor in producing energy from the sugar stores in the liver and muscle. This may be one reason why you hear many people with diabetes complain about having low energy.

Sugar that is processed has practically no vitamins or minerals. You are only getting empty calories. According to Dr. Abram Hoffer (who, with Linus Pauling, founded orthomolecular medicine) stated that when you refine and process sugar, most of the nutrients are removed. Refining will remove 89 percent of manganese, 98 percent of magnesium, 83 percent of copper, 93 percent of chromium, and 98 percent of zinc. These are vital nutrients for your life. As a result of losing these minerals in refining sugar, the body has to dig into its own stores of mineral reserves of vitamins and minerals to ensure that sugar is digested. Sugar also makes your body more acidic. To offset and neutralize the acidity, the body has to draw upon its stores of alkaline minerals of potassium, magnesium, and calcium.

Magnesium may help women with PMS (premenstrual syndrome) and it seems that a magnesium deficiency causes PMS.

Magnesium can help women who are going through menopause. Magnesium can help with male infertility, as infertile males have significantly lower levels of magnesium.

Magnesium is very vital for women who are pregnant and may prevent complications going through delivery and help prevent premature births. Magnesium can also help with postpartum depression.

Magnesium helps with arthritis. One study showed that the lower the level of dietary magnesium intake, the higher the occurrence of osteoarthritis.

According to a 2015 study in the *British Journal of Cancer*, decreasing your magnesium 100 mg a day correlated to a 24 percent increase in pancreatic cancer.

Magnesium helps with chronic fatigue syndrome and fibromyalgia. Fibroa means "connective tissue" and myalgia means "muscle pain." Fibromyalgia is closely related to chronic fatigue syndrome. Taking more magnesium often reduces fatigue.

Many people with asthma are magnesium deficient. Magnesium is a great treatment for asthma because it is an antihistamine and a bronchodilator, and it naturally lowers the histamine levels in your body. It also has a relaxing and dilating effect on the bronchial tube muscles that go into spasm when a person has an asthma attack. Low levels of magnesium increase bronchial spasms. Magnesium will also reduce airway inflammation, raise the level of anti-inflammatory substances like nitric oxide, and suppress chemicals that cause spasms.

People who suffer from Alzheimer's disease and Parkinson's disease are often deficient in magnesium.

The body's ability to absorb magnesium declines with age, so those elderly people who take pharmaceutical drugs for medicine and don't supplement with magnesium and eat a diet high in magnesium are at great health risk.

Magnesium deficiency is one of the causes of leaky gut cell membranes.

Individuals known as centenarians (those who reach the age of 100) have higher magnesium body levels and lower calcium levels than most elderly people.

The Epidemiology Journal reported in 2006 that there was a 40 percent lower risk of dying from all types of cardiovascular disease and cancer in men whose magnesium levels were the highest compared to the men who had the least magnesium levels.

Magnesium also aids in detoxifying chemicals. Magnesium helps get rid of heavy metals from the body.

Taking many drugs may deplete magnesium because magnesium is used up by the body trying to detoxify these drugs.

You lose magnesium during exercise through sweat and the rise in metabolism. Upping your magnesium will decrease lactic acid in your body. If there is a decrease in exercise capacity, it could be a sign of magnesium deficiency. The endurance of animals was restored after they were given magnesium that was dissolved in water.

Numerous studies have demonstrated that supplementing with magnesium will enhance the endurance and performance of swimmers, cyclists, cross-country skiers, and long-distance runners.

According to various animal studies, when there are high or normal levels of magnesium in the brain, if you have a stroke, the damage caused by the stroke, as well as the neurological deficit, is reduced. This is because magnesium prevents calcium from entering and flooding the cells and causing injury.

Supplementing with magnesium can lessen seizures in those who have epilepsy.

Magnesium is an extremely important neuroprotectant. It assists in protecting our cells against potential environmental neurotoxins such as herbicides, solvents, food additives, pesticides, and cleaning products.

When you are deficient in magnesium, the magnesium won't be able to do its job of counteracting the clotting action of calcium in your blood. The tiny blood clots clog up the blood vessels in the brain, and this leads to migraines. There is also a rise in other substances that assist in creating blood clots when your magnesium is low. Magnesium helps relax the blood and helps them to dilate. This will lessen the constrictions and spasms that can cause migraines.

Magnesium used to be in the water supply of many cities, but that is no longer the case. And that is one of the reasons why so many people are deficient in magnesium.

Vitamin D needs magnesium to be able to transform it into its active form. Magnesium absorption is helped by zinc.

Dr. Carolyn Dean mentions in her book *The Magnesium Miracle* that a study by Doctors Shealy and Doctor Cox discovered that out of nearly 500 people dealing with depression, the vast majority were deficient in magnesium. So maybe we may want to focus on giving people more magnesium instead of antidepressant drugs that often have really bad side effects.

Magnesium is required to produce, release, and consume serotonin by your gut and brain cells. When you have sufficient magnesium, you make enough serotonin, and you experience emotional stability and balance. However, when the stores of magnesium are depleted by stress, that emotional balance is thrown out of whack, and that can lead to depression.

Magnesium can help alleviate insomnia. GABA is the primary suppressing neurotransmitter of your central nervous system. Activation of GABA receptors will help you sleep. Magnesium will bind to the GABA gates, help boost their effects, and assist in making you sleepier.

A magnesium deficiency will aggravate a potassium deficiency. The building blocks of life, DNA and RNA, rely on magnesium and ATP (Adenosine triphosphate) to keep stable genes. DNA synthesis becomes lethargic without enough magnesium.

Magnesium helps with a whole bunch of things, such as migraines, anxiety, heart disease, calming effect on the brain, chronic pain, irritable bowel syndrome (IBS), diabetes, keeping bones strong since it helps with bone density, better sleep, heartburn, relaxing the body, decreasing abnormal heart rhythms.

Women tend to be more deficient in magnesium during a variety of periods: (1) During PMS (Premenstrual Syndrome), (2) During pregnancy, (3) Painful periods (Dysmenorrhea), and (4) During breastfeeding.

Osteoporosis is evidence of a magnesium and calcium imbalance. About 30 percent of angina (chest pain) patients do not have arteries that are severely blocked but are probably suffering an electrical imbalance that is mineral deficiency driven. Usually, the mineral is magnesium.

Dr. Carolyn Dean, in her book *The Magnesium Miracle*, mentions that 40 to 60 percent of sudden deaths from heart attacks could occur without any previous artery blockage, abnormalities in heart rhythm, or blood clots formed. Most likely, it is caused by spasms in the arteries. Guess what? Magnesium is a natural antispasmodic. Sudden cardiac death has been linked to magnesium deficiency.

You don't have to worry about overdosing on magnesium because the body will excrete any excess. You have a lot to worry about if you are deficient in it.

Taking enough magnesium to offset the amount of calcium in your body is important to avoid calcification. Normally, a calcium/magnesium ratio of 2:1 works best.

All muscles (including heart muscles) have more magnesium than calcium. If magnesium levels are low, calcium will go into the smooth muscle cells of blood vessels. This will lead to spasms, which leads to constricted blood vessels. This constriction leads to higher blood pressure, angina, arterial spasm, and heart attacks. Taking more magnesium and a properly balanced calcium to magnesium ratio can prevent all these symptoms.

According to a 2015 study, magnesium plays a vital and major role in dissolving calcium crystals in arteries that have been calcified. Calcification of the coronary artery can lead to heart attacks and strokes, and taking more magnesium can help prevent that by dissolving the calcium crystals.

In addition to coronary artery calcification, high levels of calcium without a balanced level of magnesium to offset it can lead to the development of dental cavities, fibromyalgia, muscle spasms, and calcium deposits. It can also constrict the smooth muscles that surround the lungs' tiny airways, which causes asthma and constricted breathing. Calcium overload without enough magnesium can lead to inflammation in the body. This is why it is crucial to ensure you are not deficient in magnesium. In cooking, less calcium than magnesium is lost, which is another reason for the average diet having more calcium than magnesium in it.

Unfortunately, processed foods have very little magnesium. Most of it is lost in the refining and processing of the food. When they fortify the foods with nutrients, they almost never add magnesium to the food. A slice of wheat bread will have about 25 mg of magnesium, while a slice of white bread will have about 6 mg.

If you have a high-protein diet, you need more magnesium to digest it.

People who have osteoporosis, diabetes, asthma, arthritis, gallbladder disease, and various other diseases are often deficient in hydrochloric acid. These conditions also correlate with magnesium deficiency.

Dr. Carolyn Dean refers in her book *The Magnesium Miracle*, to a paper written by Dr. Mildred Seelig and Andrea Rosanoff that demonstrated that magnesium acts by the same mechanisms as statin drugs to lower cholesterol. Magnesium is the natural way the body evolved to balance and control cholesterol levels. Statins mess up and destroy the process. If you have enough magnesium in the body, there won't be an excess of cholesterol, and it will be limited to its essential functions. Your body produces most of the cholesterol in the liver, so the body won't produce it if it's not needed. This mechanism of not producing more cholesterol unless needed depends on having enough magnesium.

60% of magnesium resides in the bones. A magnesium deficiency is a problem when it comes to bones.

Neurologist and pioneer in pain medicine Dr. Norman Shealy says, "Every known illness is associated with a magnesium deficiency." He also says that magnesium is the missing cure for many diseases.

Did you know that your body's most powerful antioxidant, glutathione (aka the master antioxidant), needs magnesium for its synthesis? Sadly, the vast majority don't know this, and as a result, millions are suffering daily from magnesium deficiency and are not aware of it. Various studies show between 60% to 80% are magnesium deficient.

Not surprisingly, since magnesium helps with so many processes and functions in the body, it also plays a role in mental well-being and brain health.

Evidence indicates that the magnesium levels inside brain cells correspond directly with energy production. It turns out that when your brain cells do not make the proper amounts of energy, magnesium levels are usually very low. Since low levels of magnesium have been found in people suffering migraine attacks, this low magnesium level may be impacting the migraine.

Magnesium has been shown to increase serotonin activity. Serotonin is known as the feel-good hormone. When the brain is deficient in magnesium, the serotonin levels have been found to be reduced.

Several studies have shown a link between low levels of magnesium and anxiety and depression. When the intake of magnesium was increased, the patient's mood improved.

A deficiency of magnesium was found in 72 percent (18 out of 25) of children diagnosed with ADHD (Attention Deficit Hyperactivity Disorder), according to a study published in the Egyptian Journal of Medical Human Genetics. The group that received magnesium supplementation saw improvement in cognitive functions. The study determined that supplementing with magnesium for ADHD demonstrated its safety and value.

A study published in the journal Alzheimer's & Dementia: Translational Research & Clinical Interventions recommends taking a large amount of magnesium daily, which can help improve cognition in elderly people.

Difficulty with memory and concentration or slow cognition can all indicate a magnesium deficiency.

Magnesium is a very important nutrient for your brain. Your brain cannot function as well without magnesium, so you should take more magnesium for better brain function.

Magnesium is very important for energy production, and it also plays a vital role in sleep.

The activity of GABA (gamma-aminobutyric acid) receptors is triggered by magnesium. GABA helps calm down and slow down your brain and helps it prepare for sleep. Thus, taking magnesium can aid in going into rest and recovery mode more easily after a long day.

Magnesium assists with regulating your wake-sleep cycle. According to various studies, your internal clocks' regularity is linked to your magnesium levels.

Research shows that people with higher magnesium levels as a result of supplementation tend to have lower amounts of the stress hormone cortisol.

In addition to helping you feel calm and relaxed and helping you feel sleepy, magnesium can also help improve your overall sleep quality and increase the extent of time you spend in slow-wave sleep. This is crucial both for memory consolidation and muscle repair.

Here are some foods that are good sources of magnesium:

- Avocados
- Dark Chocolate
- Some Fatty fish
- Grains
- Leafy greens
- Legumes
- Nuts
- Flax and Chia seeds
- Pumpkin seeds
- Raw green veggies
- Raw cacao
- Pink salt and unrefined sea salts
- Wild-caught fish

- Sea vegetable - kelp/nori/dulse
- Sprouted nuts/seeds
- Avocados
- Sprouted legumes
- Bananas
- Edamame
- Raw Dairy from Grass-fed cows

Pink salts and Epsom salts contain highly bioavailable magnesium that can be absorbed through food or the skin. Epsom salt baths are a great natural magnesium infusion therapy.

You can also take a magnesium supplement as you get close to bedtime, which will allow you to benefit from magnesium's relaxing and calming qualities.

It is best to take magnesium supplements an hour or two before bedtime so they will have enough time to relax you and make you sleepy.

Magnesium is present in all cells of the body. It is involved in over 800 enzymatic processes. Magnesium is crucial and essential for maintaining normal lung function, heart rhythmicity, bone density, and blood glucose regulation. Magnesium is a very common deficiency, and this deficiency plays a role in many of the common health struggles people go through each day.

Unfortunately, the vast majority of doctors are not trained to detect magnesium deficiencies. Since only 1% of the body's magnesium is stored in the blood, magnesium deficiencies are usually not caught and diagnosed because they do not show up in blood tests.

Dr. Norman Shealy, M.D. & Ph.D., an American neurosurgeon and a pioneer in pain medicine says, "Every known illness is associated with a magnesium deficiency" and that "magnesium is the most critical mineral required for electrical stability of every cell in the body. A magnesium deficiency may be responsible for more diseases than any other nutrient." You can sense how important magnesium is for your body's health.

Many researchers believe this RDA level of 310-420 mg daily magnesium is way too low and believe we should be taking at least twice that level. For older adults, even more should be required since, at age 70, your body can only convert magnesium at ⅔ the level it did when you were younger.

Magnesium is a very important basic element of life, just like air and water. You can compare magnesium in the body to what the oil is for the engine of a car. If you don't get enough magnesium and become deficient in it, health problems will arise.

The modern diet tends to be rich in calcium but insufficient in magnesium. Our ancient ancestors had a diet that was close to 1:1 calcium to magnesium, whereas our present-day diets are more like 5:1 and up to 15:1.

Having roughly ten times more calcium than magnesium is a serious problem and can lead to all kinds of health issues. This elevated calcium-to-magnesium ratio has been linked to autism, migraines, attention deficit disorder, anxiety, asthma, mitral valve prolapse, allergies, and fibromyalgia. This high calcium-to-magnesium ratio inside the cells often leads to muscle spasms, contractions, and twitches.

The body will have a very difficult time making and utilizing proteins and enzymes without a sufficient amount of magnesium. Without enough magnesium, it won't be able to detoxify and properly methylate or utilize and process vital antioxidants like vitamin E and vitamin C.

Magnesium is necessary and crucial for proper detoxification operations.

Magnesium deficiency has been linked to the following health conditions:

- Rapid heartbeat, arrhythmias, and mitral valve disorders
- Migraines
- ADHD (Attention-deficit/hyperactivity disorder)
- Autism
- Anxiety
- Asthma
- Allergies
- Chronic Pain
- Fibromyalgia
- Chronic Fatigue
- Muscle Cramp and Spasms
- Insomnia
- Twitching and tremors
- Swelling/edema
- Weak pulse
- Brain fog/confusion
- Osteoporosis

- Headaches
- Elevated Blood Pressure
- PMS and menstrual cramping
- Constipation and stomach cramping
- Depression
- Bad body odor
- Atherosclerosis (hardening of the arteries)
- Tooth weakness
- Vertigo

The rhythm of the heart is kept by the electrical activity of the heart nerves and muscles. The proper balance of magnesium and calcium is required to maintain that electrical activity. If you have too much calcium and too little magnesium, as is common in diets today, then the heart rhythm is going to falter. The human heart has more magnesium than any other organ in the body. That fact should tell you how vital magnesium is to the heart.

A study published in the journal *Diabetes Care* that was conducted by researchers from the University of North Carolina-Chapel Hill stated that eating a diet rich in magnesium may significantly reduce your risk of developing Type 2 diabetes.

The researchers wrote, "Increasing magnesium intake may be important for improving insulin sensitivity, reducing systemic inflammation, and decreasing diabetes risk."

At the beginning of the study, the researchers took 4,497 people who were diabetes-free between the ages of 18 and 30 and compared magnesium intake and diabetes rates. They followed up with them 20 years later. Three hundred and thirty of the participants had developed Type 2 diabetes.

They discovered the diabetes risk was 47 percent lower among those who had the participants with the greatest magnesium intake than among those with the least. As the levels of intake increased, they observed that the levels of insulin resistance decreased. Magnesium is known to regulate certain glucose-processing enzymes, and prior studies have linked higher intakes with lower diabetes risk.

Phyllis A. Balch writes in the book *Prescription for Nutritional Healing*, "The journal Diabetes Care published a study in which overweight women who consumed large amounts of magnesium were 22 percent less likely to develop Type 2 diabetes than women who consumed lower amounts."

Magnesium is the fourth most common mineral in the human body after sodium, calcium, and potassium.

- Magnesium makes and releases parathyroid hormones that increase blood calcium levels when they are low.
- Magnesium is extremely important for energy production. Magnesium activates adenosine triphosphate (ATP), the basic molecule that transfers and stores energy in cells. ATP is also known as the energy currency of cells.
- Magnesium is important for gene maintenance as it helps create and repair DNA and RNA.
- Magnesium makes new proteins from amino acids.

Magnesium deficiency contributes to osteoporosis, according to a study published in the journal *Nutrients*. Osteoporosis is a health condition that weakens bones. As a result of this weakening, the bones become fragile and more likely to break. The bones become very brittle and can fracture easily.

There are many adverse consequences of having a magnesium deficiency during pregnancy for women and their babies. Some of these include preterm labor, pre-eclampsia, gestational diabetes, restricted fetal growth, and intrauterine growth restriction.

Magnesium deficiencies cause immune disorders and raise the risk of chronic inflammatory and auto-immune conditions. Magnesium deficiencies make the body more susceptible to infection as the immune system is weakened.

Calcium and magnesium are critical metabolic minerals that are antagonists in that they have opposing actions. For example, calcium is a muscle restrictor and magnesium is a muscle relaxant. We develop chronic inflammatory problems when the delicate balance of calcium and magnesium goes out of whack. The average ratio of calcium to magnesium in our primal ancestors' diet was about 1:1. Unfortunately, today's diet supplies far more calcium and much less magnesium. The ratio of calcium to magnesium ranges from 5:1 up to 15:1. That is not good news if you want to be healthy.

Magnesium controls and regulates calcium levels. Magnesium activates vitamin D, calcitonin, and the parathyroid hormone, all of which control calcium levels. They are the three critical hormones that control calcium levels. If you don't have enough magnesium, then the body winds up, and the body deposits calcium in improper areas such as the joint, gallbladder, and arterial beds. This leads to such conditions as joint degeneration, bone spurs, and arteriosclerosis.

Many organs, not just the heart, rely on magnesium to function properly. Important organs like the gallbladder and kidneys are dependent on magnesium to function properly.

Magnesium keeps toxic chemicals out of the brain.

The government recommends taking 350 and 400 milligrams of magnesium daily for adults. Dr. Carolyn Dean, one of the leading experts on magnesium and author of *The Magnesium Miracle*, recommends at least twice this amount for optimal health. The forms with best absorption include magnesium citrate, magnesium glycinate, magnesium malate, and magnesium taurate. You can also spray magnesium oil on the skin for maximum bioavailability. Many years ago, I used magnesium oil when I suffered from adrenal fatigue, and it helped me get back to being healthy. Magnesium is truly the Master Mineral if you want to be healthy.

Chapter 32
Potassium

Potassium is another extremely important mineral essential to all cells' functioning. It is one of the seven essential macrominerals. Potassium supports the functioning of the muscles, heart, nervous system, and kidneys.

Potassium is vital for the heart since its movement in and out of cells helps your heart maintain a regular heartbeat.

About 98% of the potassium in your body is found in your cells. Most of that cell potassium (about 80%) will be found in your muscle cells. The remaining 20% can be found in your liver, red blood cells, and bones.

Potassium functions as an electrolyte once it is inside your body. Electrolytes dissolve in water. They dissolve into either positive or negative ions. Potassium ions have a positive charge.

Potassium ensures that the nerves and muscles function properly. It allows the muscles to tighten (contract) and allows the nerves to respond to stimulation. Potassium also regulates your heartbeat and is crucial for metabolizing carbohydrates as well as synthesizing proteins.

Potassium helps move waste products out of cells and helps move nutrients into cells.

Potassium will help control your blood pressure and help protect against osteoporosis. It will also help protect against heart disease and against strokes. Potassium may also help prevent kidney stones. It will also help prevent water retention.

Potassium used to be very abundant in the human diet, while sodium was not. Potassium was 15 to 16 times more abundant in the diet than sodium. That has changed significantly over the decades, especially with the huge increase in processed foods, which has stripped away most of the potassium and added significant amounts of sodium to the diet. Nowadays, the average diet has about twice the amount of sodium to potassium because of processed foods. Most Americans today get only about half the recommended amount of potassium in their diets as a result.

Food sources of Potassium include:

- Bananas
- Avocados

- Beans
- Lentils
- Potatoes
- Spinach
- Broccoli
- Oranges
- Yogurt
- Tomatoes
- Almonds
- Peanuts
- Dried Fruits (apricots, raisins)
- Salmon
- Cantaloupe

What Causes a Potassium Deficiency?

Low dietary intake is one of the main causes of potassium deficiency. Other causes of potassium deficiency include diuretic use, dialysis, diarrhea, heavy sweating, and inflammatory bowel disease (IBD)

Your kidneys control your body's potassium levels and eliminate excess potassium in urine. If your kidneys do not work properly, potassium may build up in your blood. This can be a very dangerous condition because it may cause your heart to beat irregularly or stop beating (cardiac arrest).

Chapter 33
Selenium

Selenium is an extremely important mineral.

Selenium helps with cold sores. Selenium also helps the body handle estrogen. Estrogens wreak havoc on health if left unchecked.

Selenium helps activate glutathione.

Taking 200 mcg of Selenium daily can reduce the occurrence of lung cancer by 39%, prostate cancer by 69% and colorectal cancer by 64%.

Selenium helps with Keshan disease. Selenium is a great chelating agent, and if it's in fish, it will help prevent mercury from leaking out and into the system. It protects against mercury and is a great chelating agent against other toxins.

Selenium is a powerful antioxidant. Antioxidants are compounds that fight free radicals in the body.

Free radicals are highly reactive and unstable. They are normal byproducts of processes such as metabolism that are formed daily in your body.

Many people don't know that free radicals are actually essential for your health. They do perform important functions, such as protecting your body from disease. The problem is that too many free radicals are bad for your health. Many people have very high levels of free radicals, and as a result, they often have health issues.

An excess of free radicals leads to oxidative stress, which damages healthy cells.

Oxidative stress has been linked to many different diseases and chronic conditions, such as cancer, heart disease, Alzheimer's disease, diabetes, Parkinson's disease, and inflammatory disorders.

Selenium and other antioxidants neutralize excess free radicals and keep them in check. This helps lower oxidative stress. They also shield and protect cells from harm caused by oxidative stress.

Selenium may reduce your risk of certain cancers

Selenium may help lower the risk of certain cancers. Many think it is because of the ability of selenium to improve your immune system, lessen DNA damage, and destroy cancer cells. An analysis of 69 studies that consisted of over 350,000 people discovered that having a high blood level of selenium was correlated to a smaller risk of certain types of cancer, such as colon, lung, breast, and prostate cancers.

Various studies show that selenium can be efficient at lessening the risk of cancer, death caused by cancer, as well as the intensity of some types of cancer — such as liver and lung cancers.

Since it has the important job of switching on selenoproteins, selenium minerals act in an enzymatic role that assists the antioxidants in doing their job.

Selenium may also aid in slowing down tumor growth and existing cancer progression.

Some studies demonstrate that big doses of selenium can be effective in shielding and protecting DNA, which may reduce cancer development risk and cell mutation risk.

Various studies have demonstrated that the cancer risk increases in areas where the soil has the lowest levels of selenium and decreases in areas that have higher levels of selenium in the soil.

It helps turn food into energy

The thyroid has a higher selenium concentration than any other organ in the body. One benefit of selenium is its crucial function in converting food into energy (metabolism) and thyroid hormone synthesis. Acquiring energy from food is an essential process every cell in your body needs.

Selenium may protect against heart disease. Low selenium levels have been linked to an increased risk of heart disease, so eating a diet with high levels of selenium helps keep your heart healthy.

In an analysis of 25 observational studies, a 50% increase in blood selenium levels was correlated with a 24% decrease in the risk of coronary heart disease.

Selenium may also reduce inflammation markers in your body. Inflammation is a major risk factor for heart disease.

Selenium boosts your levels of glutathione peroxidase, which is a very potent and powerful antioxidant.

Selenium reduces oxidative stress and lowers inflammation, and this may help lower heart disease risk. Both oxidative stress and inflammation have been linked to the buildup of plaque in the arteries (also called atherosclerosis). Atherosclerosis has been shown to lead to cardiovascular disease, heart attacks, and strokes.

Adding foods high in selenium to your diet is a wonderful way to keep inflammation and oxidative stress levels to a minimum.

143

Selenium helps maintain normal nails and hair. Selenium supports the regulation of iodine, which is needed by the thyroid. The thyroid is the gland responsible for the growth of your hair and nails.

Good for Brain Health and Helps prevent mental decline

Your serum selenium concentrations decrease as you get older. Minimal or deficient concentrations of selenium could be associated with age-related brain function decline, perhaps because of the reduction in selenium's antioxidant activity. It is important to maintain proper levels of selenium as you get older.

Alzheimer's is a destructive disease that leads to memory loss and adversely affects behavior and thinking. It is believed that oxidative stress is linked to both the beginning and progression of neurological diseases like Alzheimer's and Parkinson's.

Some studies have demonstrated that people who have Alzheimer's disease have lower blood levels of selenium.

Some studies have found that selenium in both supplements and food supplements could help improve memory in Alzheimer's patients.

The popular Mediterranean diet, which is rich in high-selenium foods, has been associated with a smaller risk of developing Alzheimer's disease.

Crucial for Thyroid Health

Selenium is extremely important for the thyroid to function properly. No other organ in the body has a higher amount of selenium than does the thyroid. In addition to playing an essential role in the production of thyroid hormones, selenium helps protect the thyroid from oxidative damage. It is crucial to have a healthy thyroid as it controls growth and development and regulates your metabolism.

Selenium deficiency has been associated with thyroid conditions such as hypothyroidism, autoimmune thyroiditis, and Hashimoto's thyroiditis (where the immune system attacks the thyroid gland).

Some studies have shown supplementation with selenium may help people with Hashimoto's disease. A review determined that taking supplements of selenium for three months resulted in lower levels of thyroid antibodies and also gave rise to mood improvements and overall well-being in those afflicted with Hashimoto's disease.

Selenium boosts your immune system

Selenium is very important for the health of your immune system. Selenium helps reduce and lower oxidative stress in the body. This will lower inflammation and improve immunity. Various studies have shown that increasing the blood levels of selenium in your body will enhance the immune response. Lower blood levels of selenium may cause a slower immune response and can damage immune cell function.

Selenium supplements could help improve and strengthen the immune system in people suffering from hepatitis C, tuberculosis, and influenza.

Selenium has been linked to offsetting the development of viruses, including HIV.

Selenium supplements have been shown to lead to fewer hospitalizations and an improvement in symptoms for HIV patients. Selenium has been demonstrated to be effective in slowing down the growth of the disease into AIDS in patients who already have HIV.

Selenium may help reduce asthma symptoms

Some studies suggest that selenium may help reduce asthma-related symptoms because of its ability to reduce inflammation. Various research suggests that people who have asthma have lower blood levels of selenium. Another study showed that asthma patients with higher levels of selenium had superior lung function to those with lower blood levels of selenium.

Male Fertility

Selenium helps sperm cells grow to a good size, helps sperm with mobility, and helps them to swim. These are vital factors in conception.

Foods that are high in selenium include:

- Fatigue
- Muscle Weakness
- Hair Loss
- Brazil nuts
- Salmon
- Tuna
- Turkey
- Cottage cheese
- Chicken
- Mushrooms
- Halibut
- Eggs
- Navy beans
- Sardines

- Sunflower seeds
- Grass-fed beef
- Oats
- Beef Liver
- Oysters
- Garlic
- Onions
- Fish

Signs of Selenium Deficiency include:

- Fatigue
- Muscle Weakness
- Hair Loss
- Brain Dysfunction
- Weakened Immune System
- Infertility
- Foggy Mental State
- Irritability
- Brittle Hair and Nails
- Cystic Fibrosis
- Multiple Sclerosis
- Anemia

Chapter 34
Sulfur

Sulfur is an important mineral. It is the third most abundant mineral in your body. It is also known as brimstone.

Sulfur is important for building collagen. Sulfur is required for the formation of connective tissue.

It is important for detoxification and joint health.

Sulfur can be found in every cell of the body. The highest amounts of sulfur can be found in the hair, skin, nails, and joints. Any excess sulfur will be excreted in the feces and the urine.

Sulfur is found in the organs and the blood.

Sulfur is known to play a part in tissue respiration. Tissue respiration is the process where oxygen and other substances are utilized to build cells and release energy.

Sulfur is needed by your body to repair and build your DNA, as well as to shield your cells from damage that can cause various diseases.

Sulfur is needed to maintain cell membrane permeability. This will ensure that the required nutrients get delivered to the cell and that waste products and toxins leave the cell.

Sulfur also helps with the health of your skin, tendons, and ligaments, as well as helps your body metabolize food.

Sulfur can improve joint flexibility, improve circulation, decrease stiffness and swelling, reduce pain in people with arthritis, break up calcium deposits, and reduce scar tissue.

One popular compound with sulfur in it is MSM (Methylsulfonylmethane). MSM helps strengthen the body's defenses against allergens. It also lessens the allergic response to pollen and foods. MSM also helps strengthen the lungs to deal with allergens.

Since it is an anti-inflammatory agent, MSM can also help people with asthma.

MSM may also help prevent certain types of cancer, such as breast cancer.

Sulfur can be used to treat dandruff on the skin as well as itchy skin infections caused by mites. You can also apply sulfur for acne, as it seems to have antibacterial properties against the bacteria that cause acne.

Sulfur can be found in methylsulfonylmethane, chondroitin, and glucosamine sulfate. Sulfur can be found in over 150 compounds in your body, including hormones, antioxidants, tissues, enzymes, and antibodies.

Sulfur has been used to treat many types of diseases, such as arthritis, bronchitis, gout, fibromyalgia, ulcerative colitis, depression, asthma, eczema, and constipation, among many others.

Sulfur in both supplements and topical application of MSM has been shown to significantly reduce pain and inflammation in arthritis patients, according to research by Reagan State University and Oregon Health Sciences Institute.

MSM has been shown to reduce pain and exhibit anti-inflammatory properties.

Deficiencies in Sulfur can lead to the following:

- Brittle Nails
- Brittle Hair
- Arthritis
- Inflammation Issues
- Slower wound healing
- Scar tissue
- Rashes
- Depression
- Immune issues
- Gastrointestinal issues
- Lung issues
- Memory Loss

Food sources of Sulfur include:

- Meat
- Eggs
- Fresh Vegetables
- Fresh Fruits
- Cheese
- Chocolate
- Wheat germ
- Garlic
- Coffee and Tea
- Amino Acids: L-methionine, L-cystine, L-cysteine

Chapter 35
Vanadium and Chromium

Things that are very important to keep your blood sugar levels in check are the minerals chromium and vanadium.

Insulin needs the minerals chromium and vanadium to function properly. Many people are deficient in these minerals, and insulin does not function as well in these people. Low or insufficient levels of vanadium and chromium will result in your blood glucose being converted into body fat and blood lipids instead of being smoothly and efficiently burned for energy. When people are deficient in chromium, vanadium, and other important minerals, it can lead to binge eating, munchies, cravings, ravenous hunger, and pica (eating substances with no nutritional value like paper, soil, and clay).

Cinnamon and apple cider vinegar also help with blood sugar.

Over 100,000,000 people in the United States have blood sugar issues because they eat lots of carbohydrates. Carbohydrates break down into sugar in your body. When the body sensors notice sugars, it releases insulin (which is made in the pancreas). The insulin then takes the sugars and wants to put them in our cells. It has to go through the cell receptors. There are gatekeepers of the cell receptors: chromium and vanadium. The cell receptors don't work well if they aren't there. Your body then overreacts, makes more insulin, and tries to jam the sugar into the receptors. If this continues for a long time, your receptors will get worn out, and your pancreas will get worn out. This can lead to diabetes.

Diabetes was not a common disease 100 years ago because people did not eat a lot of sugar.

Blood sugar issues can lead to a whole host of issues. They include cravings for sweets, irritability, behavioral mood swings, high blood sugar levels, cravings for carbohydrates, low blood sugar levels, fatigue, numbness in hands and feet, being tired after meals, headaches, anxiousness, waking up frequently during the night, night sweats, trouble losing weight, weight gain, sweating excessively, falling asleep randomly, and depressed mood.

Many doctors are now calling Alzheimer's Type 3 Diabetes.

Both sugar and artificial sweeteners have been shown to cause an increased risk of atrial fibrillation.

The WHO (World Health Organization) made a statement in 2003 that it was probably a good idea for people to get no more than 10 percent of their daily calories from added sugars and that they could lower the risk of getting heart disease, diabetes, and obesity. The US Sugar industry did not like that and worked to stop it. The Sugar Association threatened to lobby Congress to stop the $406 million the US gives to the WHO every year. Then, two senators wrote the Health and Human Services Secretary Tommy Thompson to squash the report. It worked as later the United States Department of Health and Human Services added comments to the report stating, "Evidence that soft drinks are associated with obesity is not compelling."

This is not the first time the sugar industry has worked hard to prevent the truth from coming out to the public. In 1967, Harvard scientists reviewed all the various heart disease and sugar studies that were available at the time. After reviewing the studies, scientists published a paper in the New England Journal of Medicine stating that sugar did not play a major role in heart disease. They also stated that the benefits of reducing sugar were too tiny compared to reducing fat in the diet and that they were of no real importance.

With this study that declared sugar innocent, they stopped studying sugar and focused on anti-fat and anti-cholesterol research for the next several decades.

Many people did not know then that the sugar review was secretly designed, directed, and funded by the Sugar Research Foundation in Washington, D.C. They paid the Harvard researchers Mark Hegstead and Robert McGandy $6,500 ($50,000 in today's dollars) to do damage control and make sure that sugar looks good or at least not bad. This was discovered in documents found by Cristin Kearns, which showed the back and forth between the Vice President of the Sugar Research Foundation and Mark Hegsted, which ended with the VP stating in writing to Hegsted, "Let me assure you this is quite what we had in mind, and we look forward to its appearance in print."

Big Sugar not only tried to control the narrative but also succeeded. Scientists researching sugar for decades could have saved many lives but instead focused on fats and cholesterol in their studies. It was also considered a career dead end for scientists.

Have you ever heard of Project 259? Most people have not heard of it. Project 259 was a series of animal experiments between 1967 and 1971 that was funded by the Sugar Research Foundation to evaluate the effects of sugar on heart disease risk. It was discovered that sugar appeared to promote elevated levels of beta-glucuronidase compared to starch. This is an enzyme that was known even then to be linked with bladder cancer and atherosclerosis. Yes, 50 years ago, it was known to harm the heart and be a possible carcinogen.

The Sugar Research Foundation ensured Project 259 never made the light of day. They did not allow Project 259 to be published, axed the project, and ensured the findings were buried underground. As a result, the focus continued on studies on fat and cholesterol instead of sugar.

It has been demonstrated that fructose and glucose behave differently in the brain. Fructose will increase food intake, while glucose will decrease it. Dr. Robert Lustig, author of the book *Metabolical and Fat Chance*, says, "Take a kid to McDonald's and give him a Coke. Does he eat less or more?" We all know the answer to that question.

Insulin is an important hormone, and we all need it. Insulin allows the body's main source of fuel, glucose, to go into the cells of the body so it can be burned. When the cells in your liver, fat, and muscles stop responding to the insulin signal, you develop insulin resistance. When this happens, the glucose can't get into the cells. The cells start starving since no glucose is getting in, and the cells send a signal to the pancreas to make more insulin. Unfortunately, this is to no avail. The glucose still can't get into the cells, and the glucose increases and builds up in your blood while your cells are still starving. This insulin resistance is the cause of so many of our health problems.

According to the largest study of heart attacks in the United States, 66 percent of heart attack victims suffer metabolic syndrome. The primary driver of metabolic syndrome is insulin resistance.

Cancer cells can import up to 200 times the amount of glucose normal cells do. Cancer growth is driven by insulin, which is how glucose gets into the cell.

Before refrigerators, our ancestors ate over 15 grams of salt a day. They did not suffer a lot of strokes and heart attacks. Why is that? It is because our kidneys are capable of excreting and getting rid of excess sodium. Insulin resistance is the one thing that stops and slows down the kidney from excreting excess sodium. High insulin levels will also raise your blood pressure (even if you eat little salt in your diet), and high blood pressure affects the kidneys.

One of the researchers who said sugar was ok and was paid $6,500 was Mark Hegsted, known for helping draft the 1977 Dietary Goals in the US, which led to the disastrous nutritional guidelines for America.

Almost 80% of people with diabetes will die of cardiovascular disease. Insulin resistance syndrome doubles the risk of getting diabetes, and that doubles your risk of dying from heart disease or stroke.

Chromium can also help with weight loss. Chromium is also known to lower triglycerides and total cholesterol in people. Chromium also raises HDL Cholesterol (the so-called good cholesterol).

Various studies have shown Chromium to make the cells more sensitive to insulin. People with Type 2 diabetes usually have a chromium deficiency.

Chromium may help people with mild depression.

Chromium helps make the cells more sensitive to insulin, which has been shown in numerous studies. People with type 2 diabetes usually have a chromium deficiency.

Supplementing with chromium also helps with glucose balance in women with polycystic ovarian syndrome.

Vanadium has also been shown to help people with type 2 diabetes and help reduce blood glucose levels. One of the common forms is vanadium sulfate. Vanadium increases the stimulating effect insulin has on DNA synthesis. Vanadium helps people with glucose tolerance issues by making the cell membrane insulin receptors become more sensitive to insulin.

Dr. Walter Mertz and Ken Schwartz isolated a compound from pork kidney in 1957. When they gave it to those who had Type II diabetes, it always fixed their diabetes. They initially named their discovery the "Glucose Tolerance Factor." Later, they called the main molecule Chromium. Mertz and Schwartz explain how chromium works: "Chromium binds insulin to cell membranes and helps regulate blood glucose metabolism in that manner."

A good way to think of chromium is as the gatekeeper. Insulin can bind to the cell walls when chromium gets attached to the cell walls. Only when this happens can blood sugar/blood glucose go into those cells. If you have low levels of chromium and become deficient in it, then insulin won't be able to bind to cell walls, and glucose won't be able to enter the cells. As a result, the cells starve for glucose. The levels of glucose inside the cells become very low or hypoglycemic. Now, the person's cells are starving for energy,

and he is eating lots of simple carbohydrates to try to satisfy the energy needs of the cells. The blood glucose levels start to increase rapidly because the blood glucose is not normally taken out from the cells and is delivered to the cells. The blood glucose might now hit dangerously elevated levels. Now the blood has become "hyperglycemic," that is, too much blood glucose. As a result, Adult-Onset Type II Diabetes begins to develop.
Make sure to get enough chromium and vanadium in your diet.

Chapter 36
Zinc

Zinc is one of the best minerals for your immune system.
Zinc is a mineral with many wonderful benefits. Zinc is an essential mineral. That means your body can't make it. You need to get it either from food (preferably) or from supplements.
Zinc is necessary for many processes in your body. They include:

- Enzymatic reactions
- Immune function
- Wound healing
- Gene expression
- Skin health
- Growth and development
- Protein synthesis
- Protection against acne
- Building connective tissue

Zinc is the second-most abundant trace mineral in your body (iron is the most abundant) and is present in every cell. Zinc helps with the adrenal glands.
Zinc is needed for the activity of over 300 enzymes that assist in many processes, such as digestion, nerve function, and metabolism.
Zinc is crucial for the senses of taste and smell. Since one of the enzymes critical for proper taste and smell relies on zinc, being deficient in zinc can diminish your ability to taste or smell.
Zinc activates proteins that are vital for the synthesis of collage, as well as the proteins that play a crucial role in wound healing.
Zinc minerals are also important for skin health, protein production, and DNA synthesis.
Zinc is important for your immune system and the development and function of your immune cells.
Because of its role in cell growth and division, body growth and development depend on zinc.
Zinc can speed up healing. Many people don't know that zinc is often used in hospitals as a treatment for certain ulcers, burns, and other skin injuries. Zinc is necessary for proper healing since it

plays vital and critical roles in immune activity, inflammatory response, and collagen integration.

About 5% of your body's zinc content is held in your skin. Supplementing with zinc can speed up recovery in people with wounds, while a zinc deficiency will likely slow wound healing.

A 3-month study conducted with 60 people with diabetic foot ulcers demonstrated that those patients who received 50 mg of zinc per day underwent considerable reductions in ulcer size compared to the placebo group.

Another 2007 study concluded that 45 mg per day of zinc could reduce the occurrence of infection in older adults by nearly two-thirds (66%).

A 2013 study covering over 4,200 people taking the daily antioxidant supplements beta carotene, vitamin C, and vitamin E along with 80 mg of zinc showed decreased vision loss and significantly lessened the risk of developing advanced age-related macular degeneration.

Additionally, in a 2013 study of over 4,200 people, taking daily antioxidants supplements — vitamin E, vitamin C, and beta carotene — plus 80 mg of zinc decreased vision loss and significantly reduced the risk of advanced AMD.

Take some zinc if you want to strengthen your immune system. A zinc deficiency can lead to a weakened immune response because zinc is necessary for immune cell function and cell signaling.

A review of seven different studies showed that zinc could reduce the length of the common cold by up to 33%.

Zinc supplements lessen oxidative stress and activate particular immune cells. They will improve immune response by boosting the activity of T-cells and natural killer cells, which help protect your body from infection.

Other research proposes that zinc supplements may greatly lower the risk of infections and support immune response in older people.

Various studies suggest that zinc treatments can effectively treat acne. People with acne often have diminished levels of zinc. So, taking zinc supplements may aid in lessening acne symptoms.

Zinc reduces levels of certain inflammatory proteins in your body. Forty older adults who took 45 mg of zinc per day showed greater reductions in inflammatory markers in their bodies than those in a placebo group in a 2010 study.

Zinc helps produce immune system cells that attack germs. Zinc supplements and lozenges may help you recover from a cold more quickly. Zinc may also help with COVID-19. According to some studies, being deficient in zinc boosts your risk of getting COVID-19 and getting more severe symptoms of COVID-19.

Zinc can help lower blood sugar and cholesterol. People who suffer from Type 2 diabetes are often deficient in zinc. A good number of experts believe these deficient zinc levels can make the disease get worse quickly. Various studies suggest that zinc can lower high cholesterol and blood sugar in people with Type 2 diabetes. Research shows that zinc may also improve blood sugar levels in pregnant women with gestational diabetes.

Food sources of Zinc include:

- Oysters
- Pork
- Beef
- Crab
- Oats
- Cashews and Other Nuts
- Chickpeas and Other Legumes
- Dairy
- Lobster
- Hemp Seeds and Other Seeds
- Tofu
- Dark Chocolate
- Sardines

Symptoms of a zinc deficiency include:

- Compromised immune function
- Loss of appetite
- Hair Loss
- Miscarriage
- Delayed healing
- Skin problems
- Pica (craving and chewing substances with no nutritional value like clay and soil)
- Diarrhea
- Loss of smell and taste
- Trouble concentrating
- Fatigue

- Anemia
- Hair Loss
- Poor growth and development
- Infertility
- Depression
- Prostate enlargement
- Anorexia and reduced appetite

These are the people who are at risk for zinc deficiency:

- Vegetarians and vegans
- People with sickle cell diseases
- Women who are pregnant or breastfeeding
- HIV infected individuals
- Individuals with digestive disorders
- People with alcohol use disorders

Zinc is an extremely important nutrient with many awesome benefits. Make sure you are getting enough every single day!

Chapter 37
Ashwagandha

Ashwagandha is a very helpful and adaptogenic herb that is best known for helping the mind and body adapt to stress. It has many other beneficial uses as well.

Some of the benefits of ashwagandha include:

- May help with reducing stress and anxiety
- May help with reducing cortisol levels
- May help reduce inflammation
- May help improve sleep
- May help with energy levels
- May help improve your memory
- May help with managing blood sugar
- May help with male and female fertility
- May help with athletic performance
- Have a sense of calm
- Help with mental clarity
- May help those with weakened immunity
- Can help alleviate fatigue and increase stamina
- May help enhance immune function
- Promote Optimal Nerve Cell Function
- Reduce Oxidative Stress
- May help with hormonal balance
- May help reduce blood pressure

On a personal note, nine years ago, I suffered from adrenal fatigue, which took a toll on me and my adrenal glands. My cortisol levels were out of whack, and I had really bad insomnia. I was exhausted all the time, yet I had trouble sleeping. I would have more energy at night than during the daytime, which is the opposite of what people should experience.
What helped me overcome my adrenal fatigue and get my cortisol levels checked was taking magnesium oil and ashwagandha. My energy returned, my insomnia went away, and I started sleeping better. Part of the reason was taking ashwagandha.
Ashwagandha can help regulate your cortisol levels, which are linked to stress. It can help promote feelings of calmness and relaxation.

Ashwagandha possesses compounds with anti-inflammatory properties, and this can help fight inflammation.

Ashwagandha also has a good amount of antioxidants, which can help protect cells against oxidative damage from free radicals.

Athletes sometimes use ashwagandha to improve muscle performance and strength. They attribute it to its purported ability to ease muscle recovery and reduce stress brought about by physical exertion.

Ashwagandha may also help with heart health because of its ability to help lower blood pressure.

Ashwagandha is also known to contain flavonoids such as quercetin and kaempferol, both of which contain anti-inflammatory and antioxidant properties.

Chapter 38
Bromelain

Bromelain is an enzyme mixture present in pineapple that digests protein. It has various potential health benefits, including reducing inflammation and improving digestion.

Bromelain has many health benefits. Bromelain may help treat several medical conditions.

Bromelain can help decrease tissue swelling, pain, joint stiffness and joint swelling that result from osteoarthritis.

1. Bromelain has been shown to restrict the ability of blood platelets to clot, which can help treat heart disease, stroke, and high blood pressure.
2. Bromelain can help treat allergies and asthma because of its anti-inflammatory effects.
3. Chronic sinusitis: Oral bromelain can decrease congestion, swelling, and other symptoms associated with sinusitis.
4. Bromelain can help decrease inflammation and treat mucosal ulcers in ulcerative colitis.
5. Bromelain cream is very effective at safely getting rid of damaged tissue from burn wounds (both second and third-degree burns).
6. Bromelain may be able to help control and limit cancer cell growth.

The scientific community recognizes pineapple as one of the top cancer-fighting foods. Studies have shown bromelain to have natural anti-cancer effects, including preventing tumor growth as well as promoting apoptotic cell death.

Bromelain has been linked to increased protection against breast and lung cancer, according to various studies.

Bromelain aids in treating digestive disorders. Since it's an enzyme that specifically helps with digesting proteins as well as helping your body absorb nutrients and medications effectively, bromelain is good to take if you have a gastrointestinal disorder or indigestion.

Studies have shown that bromelain decreases the secretion of pro-inflammatory cytokines that wreak havoc on the gut lining and reduce colonic inflammation.

Bromelain has been shown to help people with any of the following GI problems: inflammatory bowel disease (IBD), heartburn, Crohn's disease, ulcerative colitis, constipation, diarrhea, and dyspepsia. Bromelain helps support quicker recovery from injury and surgery. Bromelain is a great natural painkiller because of its anti-inflammatory properties and is a better alternative to taking pain-killing medications, such as ibuprofen, Tylenol, and aspirin.

One study found that bromelain supported wound healing and helped reduce pain and swelling following the patients' procedures. Of the 80 people who participated in the study, the ones who were given bromelain reported markedly lower post-surgery swelling, pain, and redness compared to those who were given a generic painkiller.

Another study indicated that bromelain fights allergies and asthma. Bromelain stops the growth and development of inflammatory responses that affect the airways. It also decreases allergic sensitization.

Bromelain works to prevent allergies by addressing the root causes of allergies, which are overactive and very sensitive to the immune system.

Researchers at the University of Cologne in Germany took 12 patients who had already had sinus surgery and treated those patients for three months with bromelain.

The researchers discovered that after treating them with bromelain, both their total symptom scores and total rhinoscopy scores improved. They also said that their overall quality of life improved with no reports of adverse effects.

Bromelain aids in reducing joint pain. Bromelain is fantastic for reducing acute or chronic joint pain because of its analgesic and anti-inflammatory characteristics. A research trial that evaluated 42 osteoarthritis patients who suffered from degenerative spine or painful joint conditions was published in the journal Alternative Therapies in Health and Medicine.

It was discovered by the researchers that there was a reduction of pain of up to 60 percent in the participants who had acute pain and over 50 percent in the participants with chronic disorders. The researchers concluded that bromelain showed analgesic and anti-inflammatory properties and could provide a treatment for osteoarthritis.

Bromelain can support weight reduction. Research suggests that bromelain may assist in weight loss by inhibiting fat production and promoting fat burning.
Bromelain has been shown to be effective at lessening facial swelling in people who have had procedures for impacted molars.

Chapter 39
Fucoidan

Fucoidan is actually a long-chain sulfated polysaccharide. It is found in various species of brown algae. Fucoidan is found in the cell walls of the seaweed plant. Fucoidan protects it from outside stresses. These same protective benefits that are valuable to the seaweed also benefit both animal and human health.

Fucoidan helps with eye infections. Fucoidan helps with the immune system, blood pressure, and cholesterol. It also helps with stress, healing, hair, skin, nails, and health. Fucoidan has anti-inflammatory properties and provides cancer-inhibiting properties. It also provides diabetes and hypoglycemia support. Fucoidan supports healthy weight and appetite, as well as blood clot and stroke improvement. It enhances women's hormones and breast health. Fucoidan improves men's health and aids in children's health. It also provides allergy relief and helps offset premature aging. Fucoidan can also help with rheumatoid arthritis.

If you want to improve your immune system, considering adding fucoidan to your diet.

Chapter 40
Glutathione

Glutathione is often considered the master antioxidant. It is found in most of the body's cells, organs, and tissues. Our body makes less of it as we get older. Glutathione is made from the amino acids cysteine, glutamic acid, and glycine. It is involved in many processes in the body and is made by the liver and by the nerve cells in the central nervous system. Glutathione is known to protect cells from harm and scavenge free radicals.

Glutathione will improve the activity of the immune cells, such as natural killer cells and lymphocytes, and that will help the body fight infections and disorders. The body will become more vulnerable to sickness when glutathione levels become low because the immune system can become impaired.

Because glutathione protects blood arteries and cardiac tissues from oxidative stress and damage, it may lower the occurrences of atherosclerosis, heart attacks, and strokes.

Some of the benefits of glutathione include:

- Boosting immunity and protecting the body from disease
- Being an Anti-Inflammatory
- Slowing the Aging Process
- Improving Sleep
- Reducing Oxidative Stress
- Increasing Energy
- Destroying Cancer Cells
- Supporting Detoxification
- Liver Detoxification
- Improving Insulin Sensitivity
- Helping the gallbladder and liver deal with fats
- Assisting cell death (aka apoptosis)
- Forming Sperm Cells
- Transporting mercury out of the brain
- Breaking down free radicals
- Regenerating Vitamin E and Vitamin C
- Tissue building and repair
- Making Chemicals and proteins necessary for the body
- Supporting Immune System Function
- Breaking Down Free Radicals

- Crucial for mitochondrial function and maintenance of mitochondrial DNA (mtDNA)
- Improving Insulin Sensitivity
- Decreasing Ulcerative Colitis Damage
- Can Help with Skin Health
- Lessening Symptoms of Parkinson's Disease
- Help with red blood cell integrity

Some supplements can increase glutathione levels, such as selenium, vitamin C, vitamin E, n-acetylcysteine, and curcumin. Foods that are rich in cysteine and methionine can indirectly help glutathione production. Some examples include eggs, dairy, legumes, and poultry.

Cruciferous vegetables, onions, garlic, and some fruits will help increase your glutathione levels.

Chronic stress increases oxidative stress, which may reduce your glutathione levels. Make sure to keep your stress under control. Activities like exercising, sleeping enough, meditation, praying, and mindfulness can help maintain healthy glutathione levels.

Smoking and excessive drinking can also lower glutathione levels because of the increased oxidative stress. Try to avoid smoking and excessive drinking.

As you can see, glutathione helps with so many things. Make sure you have enough glutathione, especially if you are older, since your body makes less glutathione as you age.

Chapter 41
NAC (N-acetyl cysteine)

NAC (N-acetyl cysteine) is an antioxidant that is important for your health. N-acetylcysteine is the supplement form of Cysteine (which is an amino acid). Amino acids are the building blocks of proteins in your body.

Some of the benefits of NAC include:
1. NAC boosts Glutathione Production. Glutathione is the master antioxidant; your body makes less of it as you age. This can enhance immune functions. Antioxidants are extremely important as they protect our cells from free radical damage.
2. Helps support a Healthy Microbiome.
3. Helps Reduce Inflammation.
4. May Help Improve Fertility in both Men and Women. NAC may help to improve fertility in both men and women. One study concluded that men who supplement with both selenium and NAC experienced an increase in semen quality. Because of its ability to support antioxidants in the body, NAC has the potential to help with fertility in both women and men because of its ability to support antioxidants in the body. Antioxidants are known to help protect both sperm and eggs.

   NAC may also help to improve fertility in women with PCOS (Polycystic ovary
   syndrome).
5. May Help Reduce symptoms related to Influenza, COVID 19 and Viral Illnesses.
6. Supports detoxification and protects your liver and kidneys; NAC protects both the kidneys and liver.

   Acetaminophen (which many know as Tylenol) toxicity is the common cause of medication-induced hepatotoxicity. NAC is given in cases of acetaminophen toxicity.
7. May Improve Your Brain Health. Studies have shown that people with Alzheimer's, Mild Cognitive Impairment, and bipolar disorder have lower levels of glutathione. Since NAC helps boost the production of glutathione, it may help with these and other brain disorders and help improve brain health overall.
8. May Aid in Preventing Heart Disease.

9.   May Help Lessen Psychiatric Disorders and Addictive Disorders.

10.   May Help with Stabilizing Blood Sugar.

11.   Reduces Respiratory Symptoms in Chronic Lung Diseases such as COPD (Chronic obstructive pulmonary disease) NAC can help with COPD. Oxidative stress and free radicals are known to play a role in COPD, which makes anti-inflammatory substances and antioxidants a logical choice for helping to treat and manage the condition. NAC has been shown to reduce COPD and chronic bronchitis flares.

The Journal of Respiratory Medicine concluded in a review in 2016 that NAC either alone or with antibiotics can decrease the risk of increased symptoms or worsening of conditions such as rhinosinusitis, COPD, and chronic bronchitis.

NAC helps with clearing mucus from the lungs. Because of that, NAC is also a common prescription to be used with a nebulizer (drug is acetylcysteine) for those who suffer from COPD.

12.   NAC helps Prevent Oxidative Damage and Inflammation. Oxidative stress occurs when there is an imbalance between the beneficial antioxidants and the harmful free radicals in the body. When you have too many free radicals concerning the amount of antioxidants, oxidative damage and inflammation can occur. This is one reason why it is so crucial to have as much support for our antioxidants as possible. Also, reducing your oxidative can lessen your risk of developing chronic conditions such as diabetes, infertility, and heart disease.

13.   May help with Autoimmune Diseases. Many autoimmune diseases arise because of inflammation in the body. Finding ways to reduce inflammation (such as changing your eating habits) can often have positive outcomes for those suffering from autoimmune diseases. Supplementation with NAC can also help. NAC is a precursor to glutathione, which helps reduce inflammation. Thus, it is an excellent choice for those dealing with autoimmune conditions who want to improve and support their health.

-

-

Chapter 42
Nattokinase

Nattokinase is an enzyme found in natto, which is a traditional Japanese dish made from fermented soybeans. Nattokinase is also sold as a dietary supplement to promote heart health.
Natto is rich in nutrients and contains calcium, magnesium, iron, zinc, Vitamin C, Vitamin K2, and potassium.
Nattokinase has many benefits for heart health.
It may help improve cardiovascular health and help prevent heart attacks. Nattokinase helps lower both the diastolic and systolic in people with high blood pressure, which can help reduce the strain on the heart. It may also help prevent blood clots and even possibly dissolve blood clots. Nattokinase has anticoagulant and antiplatelet properties that can possibly help clean arteries and slow the development of hardened arteries (atherosclerosis). This will improve blood flow and lower the risk of heart disease. According to research, nattokinase may lower triglyceride levels, total cholesterol, and LDL cholesterol.
Nattokinase also helps lower fracture risk and increase bone density.

May Help Prevent Stroke
Nattokinase has been shown to have neuroprotective effects, and it may also help to prevent strokes.
Research shows that Nattokinase holds promise and may help to improve brain function in people who have had strokes and in treating post-stroke cognitive impairment. By increasing the blood levels of the hormone irisin, nattokinase was shown to promote neurogenesis in animal studies.

Protects Brain Health
Nattokinase has shown promise as a potential treatment for Alzheimer's disease, Parkinson's disease, and other neurologic diseases, although more research is needed.
Nattokinase has been shown to decrease inflammatory markers and activities associated with neurodegenerative diseases.

Improve Sinus Health
Nattokinase can improve sinus health and help with chronic sinusitis. According to research, nattokinase can shrink nasal polyps and thin mucus, reducing discomfort and improving airflow. Nattokinase is being researched to see if it can help symptoms of

respiratory conditions like bronchitis and COPD (chronic obstructive pulmonary disease).

Chronic sinusitis is ongoing inflammation in your sinuses that could be caused by allergies, bacteria, fungal infections, or asthma. It's the most common chronic disease in adults. Sometimes, people with chronic sinusitis may need surgery to clear nasal passages.

Aid in Improving Gut Health and Metabolism

Nattokinase is known to promote a good balance of bacteria in our gut microbiome. Poor gut health can weaken your immune system and increase your risk of many chronic diseases.

The probiotic properties of nattokinase may boost your metabolism and lessen body fat. This can help regulate and prevent metabolic disorders like diabetes and obesity.

Chapter 43
Turmeric

Turmeric is a spice used in cooking and traditional medicine for many years. It adds flavors and nutrition to food and has been used to treat various conditions. Turmeric and its main component, curcumin, have many wonderful health benefits.

Some of the health benefits of Turmeric include:

- It is Anti Inflammatory
- Helps increase the antioxidant capacity of the body
- Can help improve memory
- Helps relieve and lessen pain
- It may lower the risk of heart disease because of its ability to reduce
  oxidation and inflammation
- May help with depression as it may help increase levels of serotonin
  and dopamine
- May help prevent certain types of cancer
- May help lessen and ease symptoms of osteoarthritis
- May help with diabetes
- May help with Alzheimer's disease and Dementia
- May help improve skin health
- May help with rheumatoid arthritis
- May help prevent Eye Degeneration
- Help Lower Blood Pressure
- Lessens Arthritic pain
- May help prevent and treat diabetes
- Can help with Weight Loss
- May Improve Liver and Kidney Function
- Can help treat Ulcers and Irritable Bowel Syndrome
- Increase Cellular Glutathione Levels
- Inhibit Tumor Growth
- Protect against free radical damage
- Helps reduce plaque buildup in the arteries
- Assists in getting calcium out of the heart muscle cells
- Helps protect against an enlarged heart
- Helps improve gut health

Turmeric helps with so many functions in the body. In addition to its antioxidant and anti-inflammatory benefits, turmeric has many benefits for your gut health.

Some of the things that turmeric does to help with digestion and relieve gastrointestinal issues include:

- Increasing digestive enzyme activity
- Improving liver function
- Improving pancreas function
- Enhancing stomach function
- Relieving and preventing heartburn and acid reflux
- Stimulating bile production in the liver and in the gallbladder
- Relieving flatulence and bloating and inhibiting gas formation in the GI tract
- Relieving nausea brought about by food poisoning
- Relieving and preventing abdominal pain brought about by gastrointestinal disorders
- Neutralizing various microbial and bacterial toxins and parasite infections to help prevent and relieve food poisoning

Larry Trivieri, Jr., in his book *Turmeric For Your Health*, talks about how curcumin can protect against cancer development and work to reverse it. He gives various examples of how it helps treat brain, breast, colon, prostate, bladder, leukemia, liver, pancreatic, and skin cancer.

Trivieri writes regarding brain cancer, "Research with mice has shown, for example, that because curcumin is capable of crossing the blood-brain barrier without causing harm to healthy brain cells, it has the ability to block the formation of brain neuroblastoma tumors while also eliminating neuroblastoma cells by inducing apoptosis. This study builds on previous research of human neuroblastoma cell lines, which showed that curcumin, in combination with resveratrol, a compound derived from wine and grapes, also induces apoptosis in neuroblastoma cells. Neuroblastoma is a particularly aggressive form of brain cancer that affects the peripheral nervous system and primarily strikes in childhood."

A clinical trial was done of 367 people suffering from osteoarthritis in their knees. On a scale of 1 to 10, where 10 is the highest, all of them had pain scores greater than 5. They were divided into two groups. Group 1 had 185 patients and was given turmeric extract of 1,500 mg a day for four weeks. The other 182 patients were given 1,200 mg per day of ibuprofen.

Both groups of patients at the beginning of the study had the same degree of pain and overall symptoms. At the end of four weeks, the turmeric and ibuprofen groups were equally effective at relieving pain caused by osteoarthritis. However, the ibuprofen group had a significantly higher number of abdominal pain and discomfort events than the turmeric group. This shows that turmeric is as effective as ibuprofen at relieving pain but is much safer and more suitable for long-term use than ibuprofen.

A scientific review and analysis of studies done on curcumin and turmeric between 1998 and 2013 and published in PubMed show both substances can prevent insulin resistance and lower blood sugar levels.

Another study discovered that curcuminoids reduce oxidative stress. That same study also showed that curcuminoids lowered the risk of cardiovascular disease linked with type II diabetes about the same as statin drugs. Statin drugs are known to have a whole bunch of dangerous side effects, while turmeric and curcumin are not known to have any harmful side effects.

A study published in Diabetes Care, a medical journal from the American Diabetes Association, showed how turmeric and curcumin can prevent type II diabetes. The study looked at 240 people over the age of 35 who had prediabetes and lasted nine months.

The participants were educated on how to lead a healthy lifestyle for the three months before the study started, including the importance of eating a healthy diet and exercising.

The participants were split into two groups. One group was given three capsules of curcumin of 250 mg twice a day. The second group was given three placebo capsules taken twice a day.

At the end of six months, 9.5 percent (11 people) in the placebo group developed type II diabetes. At the end of nine months, 16.4 percent (19 people) in the placebo group developed type II diabetes. Not one person in the curcumin group developed type II diabetes, and their health numbers improved throughout the study.

-

-

Chapter 44
Final Thoughts and Conclusion

You need to take control of your health. You can't let others take control of your health, especially those who profit from you getting sick.

Remember Garbage In = Garbage Out. If you feed yourself garbage, then don't expect to become healthy. You take good care of your car and give it quality oil and gas because you want it to run efficiently. You should do the same thing with your body. You need to feed your body good stuff and make sure that you are taking good care of yourself so that your body will run as well as that car you are taking such good care of.

Make sure to limit the amount of processed foods, carbohydrates, wheat, and vegetable and seed oils. Try to eat as much real food as possible.

Remember, while eating a healthy diet is important, you won't be able to get all the nutrients necessary to have optimal results from eating a good and balanced diet since the soils are depleted of nutrients. You will need to supplement. If you don't supplement, you will be deficient in certain nutrients, which can lead to various diseases in the long run.

Practice some meditation. You will develop more emotional control and will be more relaxed. You will see yourself less stressed, and a lot of your negative emotions will go away. You must realize that your brain is being bombarded constantly, and meditation is one way of helping it relax. Just like you need to detox your stomach, you must also detox your mind. You will also see your learning and memory enhanced when you meditate. Try it and do meditation consistently, and you will feel better.

Make sure you are drinking enough water. We are between 60 to 70 percent water, so it makes sense to drink plenty of water. Drinking water when you wake up in the morning is especially important because your body has not had any water for 8 hours and is dehydrated.

Make sure you get enough sleep. Sleep is extremely important for your health and well-being.

Do deep breathing exercises. They will help relieve stress as well as help lower blood pressure.

Start being grateful. People who are happy and healthy also tend to be grateful also. People who have an attitude of gratitude find many things to be grateful for and do not take things for granted. When you start finding things to be grateful for, you start finding more things to be grateful for, and you wind up being happier. You can't be grateful and upset at the same time.

Forgive people, and don't hold on to grudges. People often hold on to grudges that they have held for years and sometimes for decades against something someone did to them. What is interesting is that very often, the other person has no idea what they did to you. You are letting what they did live rent-free in your head, and it is having a negative effect on your health. There is a saying that holding on to grudges and being bitter and resentful is like drinking poison and hoping it will kill the other person. You must understand that forgiveness is more for you than it is for the other person. Forgiveness is freeing.

Stop worrying about things you can't control. Too often, people worry too much about things they can't control or influence. That extra stress and worry will harm your gut and your health, and in the long term, it will lead to all kinds of illnesses. Focus on the things that you can control and influence. Work on keeping your stress levels low. Stress can have a very damaging effect on your health. People who live longer state that one of their secrets to living longer is controlling their stress and not letting it control them.

Make sure to laugh every day. Children are often happy because they laugh a lot. Children laugh between 300 and 400 times a day, while adults laugh between 15 and 20 times a day. Laughter is good for your health. Norman Cousins wrote the book, *Anatomy of an Illness*, where he talked about how he overcame a devastating and crippling disease with the help of his doctor by laughing a lot and watching a lot of funny shows and movies. That book shows how powerful your mind can be when you program it in the right way. The body has great healing capabilities. Laugh more and watch some funny shows.

Spend some time in nature. You get numerous mental and physical benefits from spending time in nature. It helps reduce stress, depression, and anxiety. Spending time in nature will also improve your memory and cognition. Heart health is supported by spending time less stressed, exercising, and walking outdoors. According to a study published in the journal Environmental Health Perspectives, spending more time in green, natural environments corresponded to a decreased mortality rate of 12%. People in the Blue Zones, noted for having the longest life spans on earth, spend a lot of time outside activities. Spending time in nature and outdoors and getting more sunlight has also been shown to improve sleep quality.

Investing in your health is the best investment you can make. Don't think of your health as an expense but as a great investment.

Make sure to pray. Prayer is powerful. In addition to the obvious spiritual benefits of prayer, such as drawing closer to God, prayers have various health benefits. They include lower stress, reduced fear, improved mood, better heart health, improved self-esteem, reduced feelings of loneliness, a calmer nervous system, and reduced anger.

Stop drinking soft drinks and colas. When you go to a restaurant, and they ask you what you would like to drink, ask for water. You are getting a lot of sugar or fake sugars when you order a soft drink, and it all adds up day after day as you are getting no nutrition while drinking the soda and increasing your carb consumption. Studies have also shown that the phosphoric acid in sodas and carbonated drinks reduces bone mineral density in people, especially women. Phosphoric acid can also increase body acidity, cause kidney damage, and decrease the amount of nutrients in your body. Sodas and carbonated drinks also neutralize stomach acid, which will reduce your ability to absorb nutrients.

Conversely, while supplementing is extremely important, you can't eat a garbage diet devoid of real food and high in processed foods, carbs, wheat, and seed oil and think all will be ok by taking supplements. You simply can't out-supplement a bad diet. You will have health issues in the long run.

You also can't outrun a bad diet. Exercise is important, but exercise only factors 15-20% in weight loss. Diet is the primary factor in weight loss (about 80%). Remember to supplement after having a good workout to help offset the nutrients you lost during the workout, so you don't wind up being deficient in nutrients.

Lowering the amount of processed foods, carbs, and seed oils will greatly improve your chances of losing weight.

When buying food, always look at the ingredients. If you have trouble announcing some of the ingredients, you probably should not buy it. It has been said that if it comes from a plant, you can eat it; if it is made in a plant, you should not eat it.

Too much is focused on treating sickness instead of preventing sickness. Remember, "An ounce of prevention is worth a pound of cure," as Ben Franklin said. Preventing sickness and disease is much cheaper than the cost of treating disease when you get sick. If you don't want to pay the farmer now, you will pay the doctor later.

Try to think of your health as an investment instead of an expense. You spend good money taking care of your car and your house. Isn't it worth spending money to take care of yourself? Aren't you worth it?

I mentioned making sure to supplement. Make sure you spend money on good-quality supplements. Don't be penny-wise and pound-foolish. Too often, people find something online or get it from their local pharmacy chain and assume that their multivitamin or other supplement is good quality. Unfortunately, that is often not the truth. Most of those multivitamins have poor absorbability. They have an absorbability of 8 to 20 percent. That is unacceptable. You are throwing most of your money away by doing that. Try to find something that has a much higher absorbability rate (at least 90%). You are not what you consume. You are what you absorb. Better to spend a little more money if you are getting a much higher absorption. Do your research and find out the information before making a purchase. You owe it to yourself because you deserve it. My wish and desire were to give you information to empower you to improve your health and live a happier life. I hope you found this information beneficial.

Go out there and make the most of your life!

God bless!

ABOUT THE AUTHOR

Victor Dedaj is a lifelong New Yorker born and raised in the Bronx. Victor is a Certified Wholistic Health Coach as well as a Health, Wellness, and Nutritional Consultant. He is passionate about helping people become healthy.

Victor is also a Certified Trainer in the Success Principles and the Canfield Methodology by Jack Canfield.

He is the host of the podcasts *Value With Victor* and *Entrepreneurs Visiting Victor*.

Victor Dedaj is the author of the book *You Can Become Successful*. He is also a contributing author to Mark Hoverson's book *The Million Dollar Day: Proven 24-Hour Blueprint Reinvents Your Future With Radical Productivity, Profits & Peace of Mind*.

Victor is a co-author of the book *Success Breakthroughs* with Jack Canfield. He is also a co-author of the book *Dating Destiny* with Nate Obryant.

He is also a Global Internet Entrepreneur and Network Marketer in the Health and Nutrition sector.

Victor is also a transformational trainer, coach, and motivational speaker. He loves helping people succeed and inspiring them to achieve great things in their lives.

Victor believes that the more people you serve and help become successful, the more successful you'll be in life. He believes that you should focus on helping people. They want to know that you care about them first. Once they know that you care about them and have their best interests at heart, they will want to work with you in whatever business you are in.

Victor Dedaj is an active and devoted Catholic.

You can learn more about Victor at https://www.victordedaj.com
You can get a free health evaluation at
http://www.yourfreehealthevaluation.com

Made in United States
Troutdale, OR
07/04/2024

21008442R10104